THE AMERICAN TRAGEDY
OF COVID-19

Explorations in Contemporary Social-Political Philosophy (ECSPP)

Series Editors: Naomi Zack (Lehman College, CUNY) and Laurie Shrage (Florida International University)

As our world continues to be buffeted by extreme changes in society and politics, philosophers can help navigate these disruptions. Rowman & Littlefield's ECSPP series books are intended for supplementary classroom use in intermediate to advanced college-level courses to introduce philosophy students and scholars in related fields to the latest research in social-political philosophy. This philosophical series has multidisciplinary applications and the potential to reach a broad audience of students, scholars, and general readers.

Titles in the Series

Beyond Blood Oil: Philosophy, Policy, and the Future, by Leif Wenar, Anna Stilz, Michael Blake, Christopher Kutz, Aaron James, and Nazrin Mehdiyeva
Reviving the Social Compact: Inclusive Citizenship in an Age of Extreme Politics, by Naomi Zack
Making and Unmaking Disability: The Three-Body Approach, by Julie Maybee
Comparative Just War Theory: Beyond Hegemonic Discourses, edited by Luís Cordeiro-Rodrigues and Danny Singh
Living with Animals: Rights, Responsibilities, and Respect, by Erin McKenna
The American Tragedy of COVID-19: Social and Political Crises of 2020, by Naomi Zack

THE AMERICAN TRAGEDY OF COVID-19

Social and Political Crises of 2020

Naomi Zack

ROWMAN & LITTLEFIELD
Lanham • Boulder • New York • London

Published by Rowman & Littlefield
An imprint of The Rowman & Littlefield Publishing Group, Inc.
4501 Forbes Boulevard, Suite 200, Lanham, Maryland 20706
www.rowman.com

6 Tinworth Street, London SE11 5AL, United Kingdom

British Library Cataloguing in Publication Information Available

Library of Congress Cataloging-in-Publication Data

Names: Zack, Naomi, 1944– author.
Title: The American tragedy of COVID-19 : social and political crises of 2020 / Naomi Zack.
Description: Lanham : Rowman & Littlefield, [2021] | Series: Explorations in contemporary social-political philosophy | Includes bibliographical references and index. | Summary: "Naomi Zack presents an organized analysis of the major crises of COVID-19 in US government and society during 2020. While preparation for this disaster was lacking, we can learn from the fallout how to prepare for the next big disaster"— Provided by publisher.
Identifiers: LCCN 2020057551 (print) | LCCN 2020057552 (ebook) | ISBN 9781538151181 (cloth) | ISBN 9781538151198 (paperback) | ISBN 9781538151204 (epub)
Subjects: LCSH: COVID-19 (Disease)—United States—21st century. | COVID-19 (Disease)—Social aspects—United States—21st century. | COVID-19 (Disease)—Political aspects—United States—21st century. | Epidemics—United States—21st Century.
Classification: LCC RA644.C67 Z14 2021 (print) | LCC RA644.C67 (ebook) | DDC 362.1962/414—dc23
LC record available at https://lccn.loc.gov/2020057551
LC ebook record available at https://lccn.loc.gov/2020057552

∞ ™ The paper used in this publication meets the minimum requirements of American National Standard for Information Sciences—Permanence of Paper for Printed Library Materials, ANSI/NISO Z39.48-1992.

To Alex, Bradford, Jessica, Cloe, and Winona

"[The tragic hero is a] character between these two extremes . . .
a man who is not eminently good and just, yet whose misfortune
is brought about not by vice or depravity, but by some error or
frailty (*hamartia*)."

—Aristotle, *Poetics*

"The well-organized person is happy even in Hell."

—regendered Buddhist quotation

CONTENTS

FOREWORD

"You know, we're not heroes. And for me personally, I cringe when I hear people refer to health-care workers as heroes, because at the end of the day, what we really need is for everyone to sort of dig deep and take a look at the way that they could personally contribute to making the world a better place."

—Jasmin Marcelin, MD
(https://www.npr.org/transcripts/940115260)

The 2020 coronavirus pandemic has revealed many fault lines in democratic states around the world, especially the United States. As I write this, the seven-day daily-death average in the United States has reached 2,200, and it is still climbing. We follow the news about the pandemic, and we see a reflection of our highly polarized society. We also see the consequences of vast racial and economic inequalities for the most vulnerable among us. When this pandemic subsides, what lessons will we have learned?

In *The American Tragedy of COVID-19*, Naomi Zack explores this question. Drawing from her expertise in the fields of the philosophy of race, political and social philosophy, and disaster studies, Zack examines how our systems have both faltered and held up under the strain of this pandemic. She explores what the pandemic reveals about the current state of our democracy and the choices we have going forward to rebuild it.

Zack's book shows how different issues and developments are interwoven: from police abuse to our education system, from conspiracy theories to the culture wars, and from socioeconomic inequalities to the media and cancel culture. She synthesizes and distills the most significant moments of a year that no one wants to repeat—2020. Most important, she does this without finger pointing and shaming opponents or looking for magic bullets.

Sadly, saying we face some existential crises is not hyperbolic talk right now. Will our planet be habitable in fifty years? Will our democracy collapse? These are the kinds of questions many now ask. Under the strain of worry, we look for solutions and fixes. One of the strengths of this book is that it resists the desire to reach solutions too quickly, instead exploring the difficult choices and trade-offs we face. Echoing Dr. Marcelin above, let's not look for heroes who can rescue us (e.g., a political candidate or a new technology); rather, let us examine our responsibility for wisely choosing the remedies that can heal us.

Zack forces us to think beyond our party affiliations and philosophical camps. As she notes, she is philosophizing the unphilosophical— which means more than using philosophical tools to address ordinary problems, as pragmatism promotes. I take her phrase to suggest that we need to try to understand phenomena that resist philosophical analysis but urgently require philosophical reflection. This book will get us started with that task.

Laurie Shrage
Professor of Philosophy
Florida International University
December 7, 2020

PREFACE AND ACKNOWLEDGMENTS

This book was written while its subject matter was unfolding in the world. I would not have thought this was possible before I accepted an invitation to write a chapter for the *Disaster Law Handbook* (forthcoming, Cambridge University Press). I am very grateful to the editors of that volume, Susan Kuo, John Travis Marshall, and Ryan Max Rowberry, for encouraging me. The book has unfolded from the chapter I submitted to them, "Federalism, Culture Wars, Rhetoric: COVID-19 USA," and gone further.

I am especially grateful to my Lehman College students who enrolled in both instances of my "Disaster and Corona" course during the summer of 2020, to those enrolled in the fall 2020 semester, and to the William E. Macaulay Honors College students at Lehman College who are registered for the spring 2021 semester. I aim to continually offer this course at Lehman College, with relevant updates, until we have cleared COVID-19 from our lives or sufficiently tamed it into an everyday reality that is broadly acceptable. Not only did designing and teaching the course require that I recast my earlier work on disaster from weather-related foci to this pandemic, but it has also helped organize my personal obsession with the ongoing country-wreck of constant news and updates.

The students themselves, as scholars, activists, and essential workers—all on the front line in one way or another—have given me a sense that this work is useful. We can't solve the big problems by reading, writing, and talking about them, but we can settle our minds as we organize our thoughts. My students have ideals and are generally optimistic. This is not only because they are young adults but also because, as students, they are willing to prepare for a future that in many ways they see as better than their histories and present, even if that general future may be more impaired than the future was when earlier generations were their age. Special thanks also go to Megan Laverty for inviting me to present chapter 6, "Education," to a colloquium for graduate students at Columbia University Teachers College on November 5, 2020. Comments in that session helped my last-minute edits.

Thank you to my ongoing editor at Rowman & Littlefield, Natalie Mandziuk, who is both patient and wise, as well as consummately professional. I also thank senior production editor Patricia Stevenson. Simon Rackham has saved us all tedium with pre-production copyediting.

Naomi Zack
Bronx, New York
November 8, 2020

INTRODUCTION

From the Middle of Things[1]

COVID-19 is a global existential threat to humankind, with an epistemological dimension. The existential threat appears as a universal and pervasive risk of contagion, transmission, illness, and death from the SARS-CoV-2 virus that causes COVID-19. The epistemological dimension has mainly emerged as a battle over what counts for truth in tensions between basic scientific consensus and political superstition. The United States, with 5 percent of the world's population and over 20 percent of its COVID-19 cases, proved not to be prepared over the first ten months of the pandemic. A majority of American states began undergoing unprecedented surges in early November 2020. Many resolutely rejected adequate disaster response (i.e., wearing masks and social distancing), and if there is an effective vaccine, almost half of the American population has said they will not take it. There is an abundance of rhetoric in the politicization of this disaster, which has made preexisting culture wars even more intense. At the same time, reality catches everyone where they already were, based on prior racial, economic, cultural, and medical inequalities, as well as psychic (intellectual, psychological, and emotional) resources and challenges.

Millions took to the streets in the so far mainly expressive George Floyd/Black Lives Matter movement to reform brutal and homicidal police behavior and ameliorate centuries-long institutional racism. Others have demonstrated an inability to cope by taking refuge in conspiracy theories and protests based on individual rights according to the US Constitution. Many individuals have been isolated due to quarantine mitigation and hospitalization. Death occurs alone. A new world disorder is taking shape as the result of populism, nationalism, and opportunism. And all of this occurs on the eve of what is likely to be the greater catastrophe of Climate Change.

Yet people go on. Philosophers of current events may ply their skills toward optimism, stoicism, pessimism, or some mix of all three. The main aim of this book is to organize information about specific aspects of the factors just mentioned. My intention has been to focus on what is real versus what is part of the symbolic order, in a way that can engage the reader who has lived through the same events I have. For a philosopher, the process of organizing a cacophony of information requires not only sorting but also learning how to think about new situations. COVID-19 has been a tragedy in the United States, in the ordinary meaning of a bad, sad, and unwanted sequence of events. But, as will be evident by this book's conclusion, COVID-19 in the United States is also a classic tragedy according to Aristotle's definition, whereby protagonists are responsible for the bad, sad, and unwanted events that befall them.

The strongest lesson learned from COVID-19 is that this pandemic has revealed where we, collectively, were already vulnerable and short of virtue. Preexisting physical debilities are newly revealed, social inequalities freshly matter, and good and bad character and values are on full display. Injustice becomes evident to many more besides its victims. Individuals, institutions, and social systems falter when their weakest points implode. Quarantine and screen-centered life have afforded enough time to think and articulate ideas, which people did not have before the restrictions on movement, work, and travel kept them in place. Everything is illuminated through the X-ray vision afforded by the pandemic.

However, this is not a book about why we are seeing things differently, but rather a digest about how we are seeing them and what we are seeing. The way we see them is partly in the province of rhetoric and what we see is reality. From a viewpoint outside of a bubble, rhetoric itself is also part of that reality. The progression of COVID-19 and the mass protests and calls for police reform after the killing of George Floyd have been major events in the lives of all Americans, just as they are preoccupying news and cultural subjects throughout the world. Compassion and anger are moving multitudes. Change is in the air.

No academic philosopher is qualified to analyze such events while they are occurring. Even the most highly qualified historian might be daunted and the most qualified journalist overwhelmed. It is impossible not to get certain things wrong in the light of future events and information, impossible to avoid major errors. But because philosophers are human beings who I think have a special obligation to know what is going on, we need to build some understanding of the changes we are living through. Philosophers also have skills for putting things together conceptually, as well as breaking them down in analysis. Hence, the temerity of this book.

I have attempted to digest the present before. My published background for this book is five recent books: *Ethics for Disaster* (2009), *White Privilege and Black Rights: The Injustice of U.S. Police Racial Profiling and Homicide* (2015), *Applicative Justice: A Pragmatic Empirical Approach to Racial Injustice* (2016), *Reviving the Social Compact: Inclusive Citizenship in an Age of Extreme Politics* (2018), and *Progressive Anonymity: From Identity Politics to Evidence-Based Government* (2020). In a nutshell, in this body of work, I argued for adequate disaster preparation as a normative issue; awareness of the reality of legal impasse in unjust police homicide against innocent black people; the same justice for minorities that whites already had; the need to return to state and local government for competence and progress (given the Trump administration); the importance of avoiding backlash against nonwhites by crafting progressive evidence-based government programs to include white people; and awareness of the status nature of white racial identity.

The relevance is obvious: The COVID-19 pandemic is a disaster, calling for ethical decisions and evidence-based public policy; mass protests after George Floyd's killing are about the rights of black people to justice from the police; states and localities have taken authority for government response to COVID-19, as the US federal system allows; the George Floyd protests are multiracial, although resulting legislation may be black identity-based (which will inevitably lead to strong white anti-black backlash). This background work helps me now, but here I don't reprise it; I carry on after it.

For instance, the main theses of *White Privilege and Black Rights* were showing that black rights cannot be reduced to white privilege and that the impunity of police who kill unarmed black people is locked in place by US Supreme Court rulings, as well as police culture. At this time, in place of judicial change to curtail unjust police behavior, there is a bottom-up movement for reform in police departments, and it is necessary to recognize and assess that. The social-compact idea of the power of society apart from government still seems right to me, and the racially inclusive—that is, inclusive of whites—theme of *Progressive Anonymity* will likely prove necessary for future progressive government programs as a practical matter.

The theme of *Ethics for Disaster* was that we should prepare for foreseeable disasters. The SARS-CoV-2 virus (the cause of COVID-19) was a foreseeable disaster for at least fifteen years before it entered the human population.[2] But public health and government entities throughout the world have demonstrated an inability or unwillingness to *fully* prepare for future developments of the disaster of COVID-19, even after it hit. Still, there has been *some* preparation for COVID-19 stages, while the pandemic continues, and there is still time to prepare for future developments of Climate Change, which is also in process.

Ideally, preparation anticipates disasters such as the COVID-19 pandemic by taking measures to avoid them. Without such efforts, the best preparation consists of preparation for what is immediately forecast. Preparation becomes crisis management, which is hardly ideal but seems to be the best that can be hoped for. This will entail several kinds of response: research for cures and vaccines; prevention through disinfecting, social distancing, and masking; further prevention through containment by contact tracing; changing social habits in workplaces, meetings, schools, recreation, and leisure; supporting the most vulnerable. This kind of in-process or "live" preparation is what it means to fight and resist the pandemic. There are often-overlooked background factors, such as a certain amount of anarchy in US disaster response and recovery—which may be a factor of any disaster—and the uneven trajectory from demands on the street to local changes to judicial changes.

We also need to closely attend to an important distinction between lasting change in reality and rhetorical expression and conflict regarding such change. The 2017–2021 US president behaves as though he need only be the President of the Rhetoric of the United States, and a significant portion of the population concurs with him. When conspiracy thinking is added to this distraction, the result can be widespread, collective insanity. COVID-19 and looming Climate Change make such distraction very dangerous, because it not only removes so much human energy from effective response but also abets obstruction to effective response. Overall, Americans are in a tight spot, constrained by objectively life-threatening events, widespread denial of those events, and perhaps plain incompetence among some leaders, not to mention resource deficits. The near future will restrict us further, show the way out, or inspire some to find the way out.

This book has been written in immediate response to unfolding events, although the chapters proceed not chronologically but by subject: the virus, federalism, rhetoric and culture wars, inequalities, police reform, education, the economy, media, conspiracy theories, ethics of climate change. I found it necessary to have this subject- or topic- or category-based organization in order to process what was happening as it occurred (the mind as filing cabinet).

But chronology is also very important. I wrote almost everything except the second section of chapter 7 ("Economy") and the conclusion by September 1, 2020. My original plan was to take the results of the presidential election into account in finishing up. But as relevant events occurred, I made mention of them before November 3, using the previous practice of giving the dates of events and publications referred to in the text. Writing a book like this one in real time was challenging, and at times frustrating, but I was fortunate to have begun with conceptual frameworks that were not as ephemeral as news cycles. Still, some of this information will be outdated by events before publication. But the broad themes of the chapters should hold, as will major insights. That is my hope in scholarly terms only. It's possible that current crises will resolve and problems no longer loom, which would be much better, *in toto*. We do not know how COVID-19 will end, or when, so the ending of this book is not well formed.

I

THE VIRUS IN THE WORLD

"The way you prepare people for a sprint and marathon are very different. As a country, we are utterly unprepared for the marathon ahead."

—Michael T. Osterholm, director of
the Center for Infectious Disease Research
and Policy at the University of Minnesota[1]

The world as we know it includes both the natural world and the world of human physical and cultural construction. Natural disasters are an intersection of the natural and human world, and it is how they find the human world when they strike which produces the disaster. That is, there is nothing disastrous about an earthquake in and of itself. In this sense, disasters are *socially constructed*. For example, as Jean-Jacques Rousseau remarked critically about the Lisbon earthquake of 1775, if people had not built seven-story buildings and rushed inside of them to rescue their possessions, many would not have died.[2] The Marquês de Pombal, who was responsible for the project of rebuilding Lisbon after the earthquake, implemented earthquake-resistant construction, thus introducing the modern idea of disaster *mitigation*. At the same time, Pombal's efforts were constantly subject to political and economic influences at a time when the country of Portugal was in the process of reenvisioning the structure of its society.[3] Because so much infrastructure had been destroyed, the Lisbon earthquake disaster thus offered rich opportunities for social and economic change, especially since it occurred at a time of great national wealth.

The anticipation of economic and social change has accompanied the COVID-19 disaster, as will be discussed in chapters to follow about inequalities, police reform, education, and economic changes (chapters 4, 5, 6, and 7). Political structures and partisan tensions relevant to our own time will be emphasized in the next two chapters. But in this chapter, it is important to consider the conceptual tools for considering COVID-19, together with modifications of concepts, which are made necessary by our present pandemic.

The chapter begins with a discussion of what a disaster is. This leads to ethical questions concerning the response to COVID-19. The chapter ends with a philosophical analysis of how we can think about SARS-CoV-2, the virus that causes COVID-19.

HOW SHOULD DISASTER BE DEFINED?

COVID-19 has been a disaster, despite its differences from disasters with which residents of the United States and throughout the world are already recently familiar. What is a disaster and how is COVID-19 a disaster? Whole books and careers' worth of scholarly articles could begin to answer the first question and will doubtless extend into the future for many years, in answer to the second. And it should be added that these works extend over multiple disciplines, including public policy, emergency management, literature, sociology, history, economics, public health, and so forth. But let's be quicker. Here is Charles Fritz's classic sociological definition:

> An event, concentrated in time and space, in which a society, or a relatively self-sufficient subdivision of a society, undergoes severe danger and incurs such losses to its members and physical appurtenances that the social structure is disrupted and the fulfillment of all or some of the essential functions of the society is prevented.[4]

And here is a contemporary emergency management definition:

> Disaster: 1. A serious disruption of the functioning of a community or a society causing widespread human, material, economic or environmental losses which exceed the ability of the affected community or society to cope using its own resources (ISDR) [UN International

Strategy for Disaster Reduction]. 2. Situation or event, which over-whelms local capacity, necessitating a request to national or international level for external assistance (CRED) [Center for Research on the Epidemiology of Disasters].[5]

Combining these two, what we have is that a disaster is a destructive event, distinct in time and space, which is both physically and socially destructive, so that resources where it occurs are overwhelmed. Clearly, this won't do for COVID-19, which is global and, although it may have a beginning, does not have a foreseeable end.

At this point, E. L. Quarantelli, who wrote extensively about the theoretical role of disaster, is extremely helpful. Quarantelli claimed that problems with existing definitions of disaster not only result in new definitions of what disasters are but also enable us to expand our thinking about disaster in ways that can help us understand the conditions of disaster, which may include something like changes in mental health. For Quarantelli, if changes in mental health accompany distinct events that would qualify as disasters, then those changes are part of the disaster. This idea merges what may have been viewed in cause and effect terms, with the disaster the cause and emotional depression an effect. Instead, according to Quarantelli, the emotional depression following the time of a destructive event, such as a fire or hurricane, is part of that disaster. This is what it means to say that disaster is *socially constructed*—certain changes in society should be viewed as part of a disaster and not merely an effect of a disaster.[6]

In making this point, which is a point about human beliefs and experience, Quarantelli describes the New Madrid earthquake of 1811–1812, which affected local topography and changed the course and channel of the Mississippi River but did not qualify as a disaster, because the surrounding population was sparse and there was no loss of life or property. Quarantelli then compares the description of the New Madrid earthquake with a false story about a major dam break. Behavior after the false story of the dam break was similar to behavior after the actual Teton Dam break, so that both the false and the real dam breaks were disasters, in contrast to the New Madrid earthquake.[7]

Quarantelli offers both an emergency management definition of disaster and a definition of disaster as a relative event that may be extended over time, with different effects, including differences in perception and belief. Quarantelli's emergency management definition has a certain amount of irony and poignancy to it:

> Disasters are ad hoc, irregular occasions that involve a crisis; there is relative consensus that things have to be done, but the wherewithal is not enough to meet the demand. In a disaster, there is considerable variation in how the everyday capability/resource and demand/need balance gets unbalanced.[8]

Added to the emergency management definition is the idea of crisis attached to disaster as well as a sense of urgency that "things have to be done." And it is poignant and ironic that there is no talk of disaster if the wherewithal is enough to meet the demand! So we could add to this that a precipitating factor for a disaster is exactly a humanistic strain that focuses on an inability to do the things that "have to be done." We could say that disaster reaches us with complaint, regret, need, and frustration built into it.

Quarantelli was not fazed by what many seem unable to grasp in failing to identify COVID-19 as a disaster, because its precipitating event or agent is not distinct in time and place. He was prepared to accept a very far-ranging definition of what could be the same disaster, over different places and times:

> A disaster is not a unitary whole for different areas or communities. For different organizations and families, the "same" disaster may start and may stop at different chronological points. For example, a weather service may start getting involved in a disaster with the first sighting of danger cues picked up by its monitoring system, and its involvement may end after a warning message has been issued. In the same situation, the disaster for some governmental agricultural agency may start six months after actual impact, because certain crops might not be planted until that time due to saltwater contamination, and the organizational involvement may end only two years after that.
>
> The importance of noting this is that what is considered a disaster and its duration can vary, and usually does, even for emergency organizations which may become involved. Thus, what may appear to be an urgent matter to one group requiring immediate action, is not seen in that light at all by another organization. There are differential time involvements and differential time withdrawals from a disaster.

> A disaster is not a fixed entity out there with fixed time duration. A disaster, insofar as its existence is concerned, is always a relative matter, varying according to whose perspective is being applied.[9]

This exactly captures the situation with COVID-19 in the United States: different curves, different surges, different victims, different political perspectives, and different senses of urgency, all at different times in different places, and yet, of course, the same disaster unfolding.

In a later publication—Quarantelli died in 2017—he raised the question of whether the world was ready for a new kind of disaster, in the form of a pandemic. But as we have seen, his earlier theme that a disaster is not simply a natural entity or event, but the whole of that event and how it becomes integrated in human society, is particularly appropriate for our present situation.[10]

DISASTER ETHICS AND THE ETHICS OF COVID-19

Early on in COVID-19 USA, I was asked to answer "The Big Question" by *Scientific Inquirer*. I had not yet gathered my wits for addressing the pandemic, and at short notice, for a multidisciplinary or general audience, my answer went like this.

What is the biggest ethical question that has arisen as a result of the coronavirus pandemic?

In an ethical question, human life or well-being is at stake. The biggest ethical question resulting from the coronavirus pandemic is: How much do we as a society and as individuals value human life and well-being?

Why is it significant?

It is significant because the higher we value human life and well-being, the greater will be the economic and social sacrifices we are willing to make to preserve them.[11]

Here, I need to complicate this answer with some tools of the (philosophical) trade, which will bring us to disaster ethics. To begin with, the "we" is vague. There are many "we's" in COVID-19: the entire US population, the population of a state, the population of a city, the members of specific institutions, such as colleges and universities, members of different racial and ethnic groups, members of different socioeconomic classes and occupations, and different household units, from those living alone to nuclear and multigenerational families.

Also, it's not as though all members of every "we" have an equal say. Decisions tend to be made by leaders or those with power and authority, although individuals have some autonomy in abiding by such decisions, which depends on their tolerance for risk—that is, risk of the disease and risk of loss from avoiding it. Different perspectives go along with different leadership positions. There is the perspective of medical and epidemiological experts, according to whom an entire population is the subject whose human life and well-being ought to be preserved. And there is the perspective of political and institutional leaders who might prioritize economic concerns in terms of spending and production, as well as the preservation of the organizations in which they serve or over which they have power and authority. In a free society, there need not be agreement among the different leaders of different constituencies, real or imagined—and the first ten months of COVID-19 in the United States have made that point abundantly clear.

To some extent, incongruences within the United States are the result of a federal structure of government, as will be discussed in chapter 2. But the federal structure of government is just that: a structure that leaves the content of leadership open or contingent. Regardless of content, one thing about COVID-19 is absolutely clear: COVID-19 is an existential situation. This means that decisions are connected to other decisions by the nature of the situation or circumstances themselves, so that one has to take the whole situation into account, in order to understand COVID-19.

The situation or circumstances of COVID-19 are that it is an infectious disease that is transmitted within any given population, rather than affecting a population all at once. Earthquakes and hurricanes are external to populations as weather events. Although they affect different segments of any population differently, according to preexisting vulnerabilities, they can be said to be a shared situation or circumstance with a factor that is external to some segments of a population—if my house or workplace is destroyed, it does not physically affect your house or workplace. But with COVID-19, the mere fact of one person having it means that they can transmit it to other persons, randomly, effortlessly, without intent, and without doing anything special. In fact, it is what people normally do in interacting with others, such as talking to them when closer than six feet away, which is how transmission occurs.

This fact about the transmission of COVID-19 entails that whatever enables transmission becomes a risk of contagion. And that entails that leadership decisions immediately have risk built into them. To acknowledge the existence of COVID-19 is thereby to acknowledge the risk of illness and death through contagion. Illness and death are matters of human well-being and life. Leadership decisions about COVID-19 are thereby ethical decisions. Once leaders acknowledge the existence of COVID-19, and with that the basic facts of contagion, they cannot have any plausible deniability if they make a decision that increases contagion or fails to lesson contagion when they could have made a decision to do that. However, failing to make a decision to lessen contagion may not be as clear-cut as making a decision that increases contagion. This is because there are perennial disagreements about whether agents are responsible for the consequences of what they fail to do, especially when such consequences were neither foreseen nor intended, but rather bad luck, morally speaking.[12] It will suffice for our purposes here in describing the situation or circumstance of COVID-19 to keep in mind the kinds of leadership decisions that increase contagion.

Overall, it should be emphasized that the only way for leaders to avoid moral badness is to avoid making decisions that increase contagion. And the only way to avoid the appearance of such decisions is to appear to be ignorant about the facts of contagion that accompany COVID-19. If leaders have priorities other than human life and well-being and know that they will make decisions that will increase contagion, then the only way they can avoid the appearance of moral badness is to deny the whole situation of COVID-19 or engage in somewhat inconclusive arguments that more people's well-being and life will be foregone if they deliberately make decisions that they and others know will decrease contagion.[13]

It is in the context of disaster ethics that the idea of sacrifice remains important, but first, some general remarks about disaster ethics are necessary. Philosophers have traditionally relegated disaster ethics to a realm outside of ethics (following David Hume's claim that ethics are relevant only in normal life[14]). Or they have used disaster scenarios as test cases for their moral theories or those of their opponents, in order to draw out fundamental principles and argue for or against them.[15] But, as we have already just seen, disasters may bring with them new ethical considerations and questions, especially when there are new disasters or disasters new to particular times and conditions in history. For example, COVID-19 is not new in the sense of being a pandemic, but it is new, compared to the so-called Spanish Flu of 1918, in occurring at a time of greater international connection, faster travel, and more advanced medical treatments and scientific research.[16]

Disaster ethics tends to be a mix of deontological and utilitarian principles. A *deontological* approach to disaster begins with the ultimate value of preserving human life and imposes an absolute duty to treat each and every life as intrinsically valuable. A *utilitarian* approach begins with the numbers of group members and requires that decisions be made that have the likely outcome of saving the greatest number in a group. There is a loose and general consensus in the public and among policy makers that a deontological approach is morally preferable to a utilitarian one, and this means that in responding to COVID-19 illness, everyone who needs medical treatment, especially life-saving treatment, should get it. However, it is also recognized that shortages of equipment, personnel, and supplies can and have made triage necessary.

Triage is a sorting mechanism in emergency response, whereby those who are evidently moribund or have minor injuries are treated later or not at all, while those who are likely to respond to treatment are given priority in treatment. However, during the 2020 COVID-19 surge in Italy, a triage of triage was implemented, whereby out of those who were likely to respond to treatment (specifically, being put on ventilators), not all were treated, because there were not enough ventilators. Patients with more life-years ahead of them were given priority, and elderly patients were reported not to receive treatment. No one, from relatives to medical personnel to the public at large, thought this was a satisfactory response, although there seems to have been general acceptance of its necessity.[17]

Assuming a deontological ideal of saving everyone, what should be done when it is impossible to save everyone given scarce resources? The answer to this question depends on where leaders and others find themselves in the time span of a disaster, and, more important than this, it introduces the importance of preparation. Adequate preparation can save lives, and in weather-related disasters, it has been estimated to drastically cut response and recovery costs.

Insofar as preparation saves lives, it can be argued that there is a moral imperative for leaders to prepare plans, material, and personnel for foreseeable disasters. This issue turns on the meaning of "foreseeable." Suppose, as was true of pandemics caused by zoonotic viruses, which the virus for COVID-19 is, that national political leaders, philanthropists, and epidemiological experts sounded the preparation alarm, which they, including presidents George W. Bush and Barack Obama, Bill Gates, and Dr. Anthony Fauci, did, over a decade before the first case of infection.[18] Actual preparation was nonetheless insufficient.

Clearly it is prudent to be prepared for foreseeable or likely disasters, and the success of the insurance industry, covering loss in all areas of human life and endeavor, shows that a large percentage of humankind is prudent in that way. But disaster management preparation, especially preparation for a zoonotic pandemic, is another matter, because the only entities in a position to undertake such preparation are governments. What is the moral imperative for government preparation in this case? Remember, this would be a call to prepare for something that experts say is likely but which in commonsense terms does not appear to be imminent or even on the horizon of likely events. It would be and has been disastrous should it occur without prior preparation, but only reliance on something like the *precautionary principle* could have motivated such preparation or have the potential to ensure future preparation.

Preparation is not limited to time spans before an event occurs. Preparation can continue for different stages of the event, after it is in process, in order to meet the next stage. During the COVID-19 pandemic in the United States, this has fallen short, resulting in ongoing shortages in antigen tests and personal protective equipment (PPE) for medical personnel. The result has been crisis management of shortages and looming triage amid fears of overwhelmed hospital systems and personnel shortages.[19]

The precautionary principle (PP) is a normative principle that is not easily understood, agreed upon by experts, or widely taken up among administrators and policy makers. PP has at least two formulations: (1) Prepare if you don't know the bad effects of the event for which you are preparing; and (2) prepare if you don't know the consequences of not preparing.[20] Given the alarms sounded about a zoonotic viral pandemic, this would have meant: Prepare if you don't know how dangerous such a pandemic might be, and prepare if you don't know if your preparation will be effective. Added to this was the gaping unknown, before the fact, of whether there would be a zoonotic viral pandemic—and when it would happen. Needless to say . . .

The best ethically right course of action given knowledge of the pandemic would have been early, pre-COVID-19 pandemic preparation. Without that, the second-best ethical course would have been constant preparation during the pandemic, in anticipation of further stages of the pandemic. Neither has happened consistently or systematically. Part of the problem has been an unwillingness to acknowledge the severity of the pandemic and the illness it causes. Another part, as noted, is a reluctance to forego economic gains and livelihood. This raises the theoretical question of how to consider "mitigation" in the form of mask wearing, business closures, and social distancing—that is, ways of avoiding contagion and whether, like preparation, these are also moral issues. They are moral issues if we may not harm one another, which becomes another aspect of living through a pandemic, as will be discussed in contrast to individual rights, in chapter 2. In terms of the life and well-being of the whole population of which any individual is a member, mitigation becomes an ethical issue in terms of disaster response.

And now, finally, the importance of sacrifice. In the present context, *sacrifice* is an umbrella term for the cost of adequate and morally right disaster anticipation and response: a sacrifice of money and resources in preparation; a sacrifice of money and livelihood in lockdown situations; a sacrifice of comfort and convenience in individual isolation and mask wearing. Strictly speaking, it's not clear that these are sacrifices, because they are instrumental actions for the sake of a greater good or to obey a strong moral imperative. But at the beginning of the pandemic they seemed like sacrifices to many of us, who had a low tolerance for inconvenience. Also, if society as a whole were willing to accept severe economic loss in order to save as many lives and prevent as much infection as possible, that might be a sacrifice, because employment, occupation, property, and wealth are serious goods that many would hold commensurable with health and life.

But there are other kinds of sacrifice, which are more perplexing and disturbing to consider: people who willingly, altruistically sacrifice their own well-being in order to help others; and people who get sacrificed by others in order to protect more privileged segments of the population. The first group includes professional medical personnel who have freely chosen their occupation and derive gratification from helping others during a crisis. The second group consists of essential workers who are flattered as though they are making the altruistic kind of voluntary sacrifice, but in reality are constrained by economic need or coerced by the conditions of their employment, which they cannot themselves change.

HOW TO THINK ABOUT WHAT SARS-COV-2 *IS*

When President Trump suggested that disinfectant could be an internal treatment for the disease COVID-19, the manufacturer of Lysol issued a statement that read,

> As a global leader in health and hygiene products, we must be clear that under no circumstance should our disinfectant products be administered into the human body (through injection, ingestion or any other route).[21]

Despite such warning and its reiteration by horrified Trump critics, reports soon came in that calls to Poison Control Centers had spiked.[22]

It is well known that disinfecting surfaces removes the SARS-CoV-2 virus, which is the cause of COVID-19. The president and those immediately influenced by him were displaying ignorance about the nature of the virus SARS-CoV-2 that causes COVID-19 and perhaps ignorance about viruses in general. The use of external disinfectants removes the SARS-CoV-2 virus from surfaces and partly disassembles the lipids that hold the virus together. The amphiphiles in soap more effectively disrupt the lipids of the virus.[23] This kind of removal and disassembly of the virus is not possible after the virus has entered the human body, because it would be too injurious to surrounding tissue—it is too crude. By contrast, antiviral medications and immunological responses operate on cellular levels.[24] To say that the virus has no cure is to say that there are no antivirals that can completely destroy or deconstruct it after it enters the human body.

The chemistry and physiology of viral damage to the human body is too intricate for nonspecialists to fully understand, but we can grasp the following: A person can be infected with the COVID-19 virus by inhaling the virus through their mouth or nose, or absorbing it through mucous membranes in their eyes. Indirect infection may occur by touching these areas after touching surfaces (fomites) on which the virus lingers and then touching one's nose, mouth, or eyes. The degree of illness depends on the viral load, or how much of the virus gets into the body. Once it enters the respiratory system, the SARS-CoV-2 virus takes over cells and continually replicates itself in nearby cells. The patient's immune response can destroy the virus, but an overactive immune response can damage other tissues and even kill the patient, in a cytokine storm. All of this tells us how the virus works, but it does not tell us what the SARS-CoV-2 virus *is*.[25]

So what is the SARS-CoV-2 virus? It has been called "the invisible enemy" and victory over it has been called "killing" it. But the SARS-CoV-2 virus, while not visible to the naked eye, is not invisible, because its genome has been sequenced and it can be identified chemically and through electron microscopes. Furthermore, the virus is not a fully living thing, so it cannot be killed! But it can be dismantled or otherwise destroyed. It can be blocked from latching onto cells. That is, insofar as there is no cure for the disease COVID-19, the antivirals in use do not kill it, but rather partly block its effect on cells in the body; other drugs can partly regulate the immune response; and still others address damage caused by the effect of the virus and immune reaction on parts of the body.[26] The SARS-CoV-2 virus cannot infect people if people do not come in contact with it, so it is passive; in addition, it will self-destruct over time, without a living host, which is to say that it is parasitic.[27]

SARS-CoV-2 is a single-strand positive RNA virus.[28] Its RNA or genetic material is used to duplicate itself, and it can do that with proteins in human cells, after it has latched onto certain receptors in those cells.[29] Once it replicates in one cell, it can travel to neighboring cells and onward from them. As a result, the cells and tissues and organs in which SARS-CoV-2 is replicating cannot perform their normal functions.

The RNA of SARS-CoV-2 is remarkably like the code in computer viruses. Both SARS-CoV-2 and computer viruses are sequences of information (the one biological, the other electronic), and both are already designed to replicate themselves in the right hosts (the one humanly designed, and the other a result of biological evolution).[30] Both the SARS-CoV-2 virus and computer viruses have a range of effects on their hosts, from minor changes to total destruction of their functioning or, in the case of human beings, death.

A computer virus code is designed to replicate itself within a computer program, and it can be sent from computer to computer. As the cybersecurity company Norton puts it,

> A virus operates by inserting or attaching itself to a legitimate program or document that supports macros in order to execute its code. In the process, a virus has the potential to cause unexpected or damaging effects, such as harming the system software by corrupting or destroying data.[31]

(A macro or macroinstruction is code or a program that specifies how input to the computer is related to output.[32])

We can better understand the virus that causes COVID-19 if we think about it like a computer virus. This analogy would not be useful or necessary if we already understood the virus causing COVID-19, or viruses in general. The analogy is more than a matter of comparing strategies for avoiding SARS-CoV-2 and computer viruses, as has already been suggested in college classrooms—for example, when COVID-19 began to affect student attendance in a computer science course at Elon University.[33] More fundamentally, as a matter of what SARS-CoV-2 is, and not only how people react to the risk of disease, what philosophers would call the ontology or metaphysics of the two is similar.

According to a *functionalist* view of mental states, some philosophers believe it is a mistake to seek what mental states are made up of. Rather, functionality holds that mental states are the role they play in relation to the rest of the human organism and how it behaves.[34] According to this metaphysical view, anger, for example, is nothing but certain changes in the angry person's body and what they do. Viruses in both living hosts and computers are purely functional in this sense. What they do and their effects on hosts are the full meaning of the scraps of RNA or code that physically identifies them to specialists who detect them.

In sum, SARS-CoV-2 is to human beings as viruses are to computers.

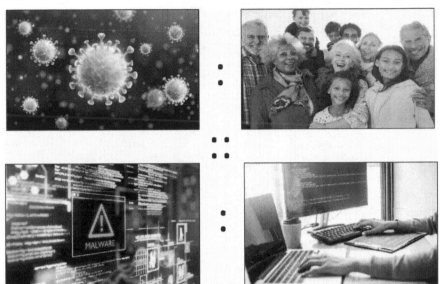

Figure 1.1.   As viruses are to humans, so are computer viruses to computers. (iStock Credits [left to right, top to bottom]: fotomay, monkeybusinessimages, solarseven, Chalirmpoj Pimpisarn)

Of course, the idea of computer viruses came from ideas of human viruses in general, as diseases that took over cells. This analogy thus circles back to its origin, but with the comparisons vice versa: A computer virus is to computers as a biological virus is to people.

Now, we already know more about computer viruses and how to guard against them than we do about viruses in general, or SARS-CoV-2, specifically. Indeed, the industry devoted to antivirus protection and cybersecurity has an estimated annual global price tag of US $23 billion.[35] By comparison, the United Nations estimate of the cost of a global response plan to combat COVID-19 is US $7 billion. Our electronic devices have more than ever become extensions of our minds/brains/bodies during the COVID-19 pandemic, but the cost of undervaluing the security of minds/brains/bodies may be prohibitive.

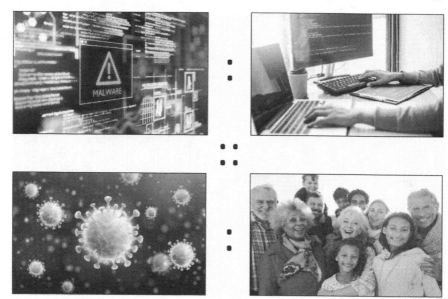

Figure 1.2. As computer viruses are to computers, so are viruses to humans. (iStock Credits: [left to right, top to bottom] solarseven, Chalirmpoj Pimpisarn, fotomay, monkeybusinessimages)

In 2018, a panel of experts was asked by the World Health Organization (WHO) to catalog known disease threats. They included Ebola, SARS, Zika, Rift Valley fever, and an unknown that they called "Disease X." Disease X turned out to be COVID-19. Dr. Peter Daszak and his team at EcoHealth were reported in *The Economist* in June 2020 as having proposed to the Global Virome Project an effort to read out the genomes of millions of unknown viruses, throughout the world. That research would be followed by a surveillance system to detect and diagnose new illnesses among people who live in close proximity to wild animals and birds that could be sources of spillover zoonotic viruses. The cost of this genome sequencing would be about $4 billion, and 70 percent of the data could be collected for about $1 billion. But "no funding bodies have yet taken the bait."[36] (This project will be discussed again in chapter 10.)

2

FEDERALISM AND LOCALISM

"The nine most terrifying words in the English language are: I'm from the government and I'm here to help."
 —President Ronald Reagan, 1986 statement[1]

"I believe we need to attract a new generation of the best and brightest to public service and I believe that government can be a source of inspiration, not degradation."
 —Andrew Cuomo[2]

In the Middle Ages, poor people over their lifetimes rarely traveled more than ten or fifteen miles from where they were born, although middle and affluent classes traveled farther and more frequently for trade, war, and political, religious, and social activity. Before COVID-19 in highly developed countries, while the poor were still less likely to travel, middle-class and affluent people routinely traveled, for study, for work, to visit friends and family, or just for recreation.[3] Moving from one state to another is often a condition for upward mobility; many own cars, which are a necessity in suburban and rural areas. Americans have taken their mobility for granted and foreign travel is a symbol of privilege, now temporarily curtailed after the European Union omitted travelers from the United States among those to be admitted in lifting COVID-related travel bans.[4]

Not only do middle- and affluent-class Americans normally practice constant physical mobility and take it for granted, but they do so without understanding how they and those less advantaged are dependent on collective goods and services. For example, as pandemic cases and deaths began to rise in New York City, many rich people fled to their summer homes in the Hamptons, the South Fork of Long Island. These disaster refugees came with money to spend on their comfort, oblivious to the needs and limited food, household, and medical supplies and services among the year-round inhabitants who worked for them during normal summer seasons. They assumed that the hospitals were at their disposal and soon emptied local supermarket shelves. They offended the local residents by partying in crowds in local night spots. So obnoxious were they that irate locals put out a call to "Blow up the bridges!"[5]

It did not occur to these wealthy invaders that they were going to a place with structured supply chains and limited resources that their arrival would deplete. It did not occur to them that they were not welcome, or they may not have cared. They used their money to escape, but it also probably did not occur to them that even their money— including electronic access to it and their purchasing power, as well as electronic connections to everyone they wished—was and is a resource embedded in an interconnected societal economic system. What would happen to the assets of wealthy people if the majority of them thought they could safely remove themselves from conditions of personal peril without taking responsibility for the infrastructures and broad economic functioning that support money as a medium for the exchange of goods and services? That is, the privilege of mobility requires that some remain in the same place, and wealth itself is part of a broad network of transactions that require societal stability.

The federal government rules over all US residents everywhere, but the powers of state and local governments over their jurisdictions are often ill understood. The bumper sticker "Think Globally, Act Locally" is a progressive call for both preexisting cosmopolitanism and new consumer attention to the city, town, and county where a person may live. In reality, there are ongoing ways in which acting or not acting locally is not a matter of choice or limited to the choice of consumer items and services. People who are not local cannot act locally without the support of the locals, and the locals may have no choice but to act and choose locally. Money is fungible, but where and how it is spent is not.

The US federal system of government allows for strong state rule within state jurisdictions. More particularly than this, residents are subject to rules and laws in municipalities and townships. We may not notice this structure in normal, affluent life, but disasters bring it into high relief. Restrictions on travel and quarantine during the COVID-19 pandemic have reinforced immobility according to preexisting structures. In addition to immobility, the local empowerment and jurisdictions of police departments in the United States complicate the practicality of national police reform, which will be the subject of chapter 5. The aim of this chapter is, first, to examine the US federal–state structure, which gives states ultimate powers in disasters and public health. Second, in the context of COVID-19, it makes sense to consider several limits to states' rights in this disaster, with a focus on the importance of local rule in terms of the pandemic. And, finally, the idea of positive rights and progressive constitutionalism merits consideration in the context of COVID-19, given state demands for stronger federal government response and protest calls for police reform and social justice.

US FEDERALISM

The government of the United States is a federal system. It is therefore important to understand the legalities of US federalism and how they have been applied in the current crisis. No two forms of federalist governmental structure are the same. For example, the US Constitution gives the federal government limited powers and reserves the rest to state governments, while in Canada, the provinces have limited powers and the reserve is with the national government.[6] Still, the constitutional division of state and federal powers in the United States does not fall into neat divisions, because there is considerable overlap. The structure of rule is less like a layer cake and more like a marble cake, according to metaphors that theorists of government have used.[7] In ordinary life, the rhetoric of national politics may make it seem as if the United States is more of a coherent whole than it is in reality. Calls for national unity, while laudatory, may be impossible to fulfill outside of rhetoric, because the general structure of US federalism does not usually guarantee or even facilitate practical national unity, as evident in the present disaster. Also, COVID-19 has revealed how the federal structure limits the power of the federal government in a disaster, because matters of public health do ultimately fall under the jurisdiction of the states.

The dynamics of COVID-19 have played out in tensions between national and state governments. Traditionally, based on the Constitution, states have pulled away from rule by the federal government, in favor of exercising their own rights and powers. From the early nineteenth century on, this has been especially true of conservative and Southern states and was often lined up with resistance to the power of the US Supreme Court.[8] But during the early days of the COVID-19 pandemic, some Democratic and progressive Republican state governors called for stronger federal measures and leadership, from both Congress and President Trump.[9]

By the time of discussion and action toward reopening the US economy, following periods of quarantine, progressive states with large minority populations began to reassert their rights. The pivot was evident after President Trump instituted militant action against peaceful demonstrators demanding police reform after George Floyd's killing. On June 1, 2020, US Park Police and members of the National Guard brutally cleared a path so that Trump could walk to St. John's Church from the White House, to make a speech, holding a Bible.[10] Although this was not military action involving the US armed forces—because Trump did not have the power to invoke that—Trump was accompanied by General Mark A. Milley, chairman of the US military Joint Chiefs of Staff, who wore battle gear. But General Milley subsequently apologized and reaffirmed that the US military had no place in civilian politics.[11]

In addition to the range of federal–state power during COVID-19, the crisis has revealed anomalies in the US system that may be more important than previously thought. To continue with the same example, after Trump's declarations about the need to "dominate the streets" so as to secure them from antiracist protesters who were demanding police reform, he ordered the National Guard into Washington, DC. He could do that because Washington, DC, is a district under the jurisdiction of the federal government and not a state (that is, President Trump is in effect the governor of Washington, DC). The mayor of Washington, DC, immediately requested him to withdraw the National Guard troops.

Two days later, after the largest protest so far, Trump had the National Guard troops removed from Washington, DC.[12] If Trump was acceding to the mayor's request, he was treating Washington, DC, as an independent state and not merely a district under federal control, although he may have removed the troops for other reasons. At any rate, the federally ordered occupation of Washington, DC, against the mayor's wishes, struck many as an unlawful use of federal power. Because a district has less power than a state, Trump's action of troop removal following the demand of the city mayor of Washington, DC, attracted political attention to the status of Puerto Rico, which is also a federal district. More to the point, the DC occupation and removal inspired a Democratic-controlled House bill to make Washington, DC, a state. Both Trump and Senate Republicans made their opposition clear, but the initiative could be continued when the political balance shifts.[13]

Thus, there was a time when, for the sake of public health, some states called for central rule by the US federal government, in order to lessen the impact of COVID-19. But after the public health crisis stabilized, or people got used to it, or Black Lives Matter protests occurred in every state and the Capitol District following George Floyd's killing, the more traditional states versus federal government tension returned. However, the historical twist of the more liberal states asserting their rights was a reversal of the traditional lineup. Overall, the complexities of US federalism merit special consideration in terms of the COVID-19 disaster. It makes sense to focus now on the US Constitution, the Stafford Act, and the history and current action of the CDC (Centers for Disease Control and Prevention), in relation to the current crisis. Discussion of tensions between state and local governments will follow.

The US Constitution

The US Constitution provides for the people's right to assemble. But that is a freedom of expression, closely connected to freedom of speech. It is not the people's right to have their views and expressive actions heard and recognized by officials in power, or their right to have their demands implemented. Policies have in the past been designed and legislated from such demands, but only if it becomes a matter of political self-interest, as well as moral principle, to do that. If there is new national policy pertaining to police reforms, it will strengthen the federal government and bypass the states, allowing for many conservative states to resist it, as they did during and after the pro-integration legislation of the civil rights movement. Without new federal policy after such robust expression of public will, states may continue to go their own way, with or without police reform.

While it is tempting at this point to consider the difficulties of police reform and the injustice making it necessary, this topic will be deferred until chapter 5. Here, it is important to remember that the George Floyd protests arose in the wider context of COVID-19 that is still unfolding. State power is permanent, regardless of the content of politics. If liberal and progressive states can assert their rights against a more conservative federal government, then, should the federal government become liberal and progressive, the conservative states will likely return to their traditional roles in tension with the federal government.

The idea that the United States is divided into red and blue states that have taken different ideological positions in approaching COVID-19 might be a good way to understand American culture, but it fails to recognize the more fundamental division between the federal government and states and the perhaps even necessary tension between them. Red and blue America may have different experiences of COVID-19 illness and death at any given time, due to differences in population density, mitigation, and testing. Such differences easily become politicized if low infection and death are lined up with the distrust of science more prevalent in Red America and high infection and death line up with high population density in more science-trusting Blue America. That lineup was evident in the early months of the pandemic in the United States,[14] and it politicized mitigation measures during the spring of 2020, especially concerning whether to wear masks.[15]

But what is true at any one time is not necessarily generally true. The Red–Blue lineup is contingent on how fast the virus is spreading, where it is spreading, and how it is being addressed there. Hospitals can just as easily be overrun in Red, as Blue, America. At any given time, the virus is always local and can only be officially addressed with ultimate legal power, on a state level. This condition can put any state at odds with the federal government, at any time, and there is nothing unusual about this structure, once US federalism has been accepted as inherently oppositional in its constitutional structure. But in its political structure, the United States has been remarkably consistent throughout COVID-19 in 2020. Republican state governors who began by opposing mask-wearing mandates—for instance, in North Dakota and South Dakota—did not change their positions in the face of a surge in cases in September 2020.[16]

A large number of rulings, documents, and organizations provide for the role of the federal government in a pandemic, in two main ways: coordination of disaster response measures within the federal government and between the federal government and the states; and federal assistance to the states in their disaster-related efforts.[17] However, in the early months of the COVID-19 pandemic, actions taken under the Stafford Act and efforts of the CDC have been most prominent.

The Stafford Act

The Robert T. Stafford Disaster Relief and Emergency Assistance Act (42 U.S.C. §§ 5121-5207) provides for the contingencies of US federalism in times of disaster by specifying coordination between the US president and state governors to deal with emergencies and disasters. The Stafford Act provides for two types of declarations from the president concerning federal government assistance to state and local governments and individuals. The president declares an emergency if federal assistance is needed to supplement state and local efforts, and the president declares a major disaster if major disaster assistance is required. Both declarations are based on requests from state governors and a determination that disaster response exceeds what states or localities are able to provide. Beyond a cap of $5 million for any single disaster, congressional approval is required.[18] On March 13, 2020, President Trump invoked section 501(b) of the Stafford Act to make an emergency declaration due to the COVID-19 pandemic. He closed by saying that a Declaration of Major Disaster according to the Stafford Act, section 401(a), might be "appropriate" in the future, should the states request it.[19]

As of this writing (November 7, 2020), Trump has not made a Declaration of Major Disaster. However, Fox News reported that President Trump had made a Declaration of Major Disaster based on section 401(a) in reporting his invocation of 501(b).[20] This may have been a simple error or support of Trump's rhetorical boosting (i.e., boasting) of his own leadership. At any rate, Trump's presidential actions concerning COVID-19 have been well within the moderate provisions of the Stafford Act, and the Stafford Act centers governmental disaster action on efforts by the states. Trump's Declaration of Emergency enabled him to draw on 136 statutory powers, of which many would say he has not made extensive use. For instance, he has not made full use of the Defense Production Act (DPA) to order companies to produce medical supplies needed during the pandemic.[21] Early on in the pandemic, President Trump had rhetorically declared war against COVID-19, calling himself a wartime president against "the invisible enemy," as discussed in chapter 1. This cartoonish turn of phrase ignored the facts that the genome of the virus had already been sequenced and that the virus itself was visible through chemical reactions and electron microscopes. Vice President Mike Pence used the same phrase when he took over the Coronavirus Task Force.[22] Of course, what they meant was that the virus is not visible to the naked eye, but their word choice could have been criticized as symbolic of a deeper departure from reality (although it fell under the radar for most critics). Still, a real wartime president would have been less diffident about deploying the DPA.

The CDC

The US Centers for Disease Control and Prevention (CDC) was founded under its present name in 1992, taking over from the Center for Disease Control by an act of Congress. The CDC is a US federal agency under the Department of Health and Human Services. The CDC and its parent organizations have always been located in Atlanta, Georgia, because the project of a national health center grew out of World War II efforts to eradicate malaria that had been prevalent throughout the US South. The stated aims of the CDC have always been lofty, now encompassing international coordination, research, education, disaster preparedness, and disease prevention, including immunization. The 2018 CDC FY budget was $11.1 billion, and its 15,000 employees occupy the central and regional offices. CDC director Robert R. Redfield, MD, an AIDS expert, was appointed by President Trump in March 2018.

The CDC is well known for its "Yellow Book," *Health Information for International Travel*, which provides three levels of "watch," "alert," and "warning."[23] However, the moral and practical reputation of the CDC was tarnished for decades before the current COVID-19 crisis, due to harmful actions and mistakes, including denying the risk of lead contamination in Washington, DC, drinking water; taking over the 1932–1972 Tuskegee study of untreated syphilis in black males who had not given their consent; promoting harmful policies for HIV-positive people and misinforming the public about that disease; ineffectively communicating information about the 2001 anthrax attacks to the public; ineffective or obstructive measures concerning gun control; and sending deadly infectious disease samples to Iraq during the 1980s.[24]

Although the CDC is primarily a research and advisory body, its response to the COVID-19 pandemic has nonetheless been disappointing, as captured in the title of this *New York Times* article:

> "They Let Us Down": 5 Takeaways on the C.D.C.'s Coronavirus Response: Early mistakes in testing, aging data systems, clashes with President Trump and an overly cautious culture shook confidence in the nation's premier public health agency.

The CDC's mistakes in the COVID-19 pandemic have included: faulty screening of thousands of Americans returning from China after the Trump Travel Ban in early February 2020; early testing mistakes and faulty tests; failure to provide timely records of infections and deaths; faulty communications with state and local officials; and not providing adequate, detailed guidance to states and hospitals. The CDC takes no direct action itself and has no powers of enforcement for its advice. But even as an advisory and informational agency, the CDC has not emerged as "the reliable go-to place," according to Dr. Ashish Jha, director of the Harvard Global Health Institute.[25]

The role of the CDC was obscured in the White House response to COVID-19. On January 29, 2020, President Trump convened the White House Coronavirus Task Force and later reorganized it under the leadership of Vice President Mike Pence. This task force provided information about the progression of COVID-19. It has issued mitigation advisory directives, including a thirty-day nationwide lockdown in April and May, and reported federal government efforts to support state efforts regarding the pandemic. The task force has been criticized as an instrument for the president's self-promotion. But at the same time, two members of the task force with extensive scientific expertise, doctors Deborah Birx (United States Global AIDS Coordinator and White House Coronavirus Response Coordinator) and Anthony Fauci (director of the National Institute of Allergy and Infectious Diseases), appear to have strong credibility among the US public, especially Dr. Fauci.[26] (The National Institute of Allergy and Infectious Diseases [NIAID] is one of the twenty-seven institutes and centers that make up the National Institutes of Health [NIH], which is an agency of the US Department of Health and Human Services [HHS], although Alex Azar, the head of HHS and initial head of the task force, has not played a visibly prominent public role on the task force.) Furthermore, the Trump administration's task force apparently encroached on the informational role of the CDC in its directive that people without COVID-19 symptoms who had been in contact with those with the disease did not require testing if they had no symptoms. Medical experts found this directive concerning, because it is known that asymptomatic people may both have and transmit the SARS-CoV-2 virus.[27] The CDC consequently posted guidelines for testing asymptomatic people.[28]

The Food and Drug Administration (FDA) will have an important regulatory role in SARS-CoV-2 vaccine distribution. It is noteworthy and encouraging that in early October 2020, the FDA resisted the Trump administration's pressure to approve a vaccine before Election Day. Instead, the FDA released guidelines requiring comprehensive testing for safety before a vaccine could be released for emergency use. Although the Trump administration held up release of these guidelines for two weeks, they eventually approved their release.[29]

This failure of the US (and, some would say, thereby the global) infectious disease leadership organization not only was an international disappointment but also highlights the US federal structure of the current crisis. The need for states and localities to rely on their own data and resources has proved vital. There has been similarity in mitigation, containment, and treatment measures, as well as mutual aid, among the states, much of it in implementation of the Emergency Management Assistance Compact that was ratified by Congress in 1996 and since then implemented in state legislation.[30] Such federally enabled but state-implemented efforts may add up to a national response or approach to COVID-19, but that is not the same thing as an effective, cohesive, national approach coming from the federal government. The pluralistic or fragmented (take your pick) practical situation is emphasized by the absence of unifying national rhetoric.

LIMITS TO STATES' RIGHTS IN COVID-19

States have rights against the federal government and rights against one another. This structure implies that if a state overreaches, it can be checked by the federal government, or by another state, or again by the federal government that has various powers for regulating interstate commerce, which states do not have. Compliance with various state and federal directives, as well as state–state and state–federal tensions and disagreements can in principle be resolved according to the US Constitution Commerce Clause (Article 1, Section 8, Clause 3), which gives Congress the right to "regulate Commerce with foreign Nations, and among the several States, and with the Indian Tribes." In normal times, the US Supreme Court has interpreted this clause by restricting the power of states to prevent individuals from moving freely among states and visiting states other than their state of residence, and states may not discriminate against individuals from out of state. Nevertheless, the US Supreme Court has in the past upheld state quarantine laws and recognized states' police powers in matters of public health.[31] The two judicial strains of individual freedom to travel and states' powers to restrict travel for a compelling interest in public health may force further judicial rulings as the present pandemic progresses.

US Supreme Court Justice Louis Brandeis (1856–1941) may seem apposite to quote in regard to US federalism, when he approvingly referred to the states as laboratories for "novel social and economic experiments."[32] There is a difference between practices within states that other states might try to duplicate and practices within states in which states or their residents have conflicting interests. But, of course, if states begin to "one up" each other in travel restriction practices, the laboratory model would, unfortunately, apply—if it were effective in keeping low-infection areas low. The laboratory model might also apply, albeit inadvertently. For instance, states that have reopened quickly and then closed down again might have different economic and disease data compared to states that were more cautious in reopening or never even closed down.[33] If, depending on their public health and economic priorities, states learn from one another, either by doing what other states have done or by deliberately avoiding what other states have done, then such inadvertent experimentation might have long-term benefits.

Insofar as citizen well-being, and with that, disaster response, is within the authority of states, so far during the COVID-19 pandemic, there have been tensions between states and the federal government and states and states. However, a couple of advisory-type states' rights assertions by state governments are worth noting. In March 2020, while New York was experiencing its surge in COVID-19 cases, the governors of both Florida and Rhode Island spoke of directives that travelers from New York should quarantine upon arrival or else be refused entry. New York's Governor Cuomo vigorously opposed these measures and said he would take them to court. Both states stood down.[34] But in June 2020, when there were surges in Southern and Western states, New York issued an advisory directive that travelers from high-surge states quarantine for fourteen days upon arrival to New York.[35] It was not made clear to what extent this directive was an "honors system" or a real rule that would be punitively enforced. The advisory nature of these travel restrictions reflects the generally cooperative attitude of state governments toward each other during this pandemic, as well as the likelihood that laws restricting interstate travel or commerce might not withstand judicial review for constitutional reasons.

State–federal and state–state government conflicts are not the whole story. COVID-19 has brought out citizen–state and locality–state conflicts over responses to the pandemic, responses that are deeply rooted in opposing philosophies and activism. Saying that governors have been the primary leaders in COVID-19 response does not mean that they have had the resources or political support within their own states to either carry out effective measures against the virus or reopen businesses. Outcomes depend on politics within states, on whether a governor has the support of the opposing political party in a state legislature or whether local leaders believe that state policies meet their pandemic needs.

Governor Gretchen Whitmer of Michigan, a Democrat in a state with a gerrymandered Republican-controlled legislature, was elected to office in 2018 during the midterm elections that were overall successful for Democrats. Whitmer was unable to get adequate supplies in the early days of the pandemic, because, like other US state governors, she had to compete for personal protective equipment (PPE) and ventilators against the federal government in global markets. (It was apparently not unusual for the federal government to commandeer supplies purchased by states while they were en route to their buyers.) Many assumed that the Strategic National Stockpile was a resource for the states, but the president's son-in-law, Jared Kushner, who set up a kind of "shadow" Coronavirus Task Force to supplement the official one, sought to disabuse Americans of that notion. He proclaimed:

> You also have a situation where in some states, FEMA allocated ventilators to the states and you have instances where in cities they're running out, but the state still has a stockpile and the notion of the federal stockpile was, it's supposed to be our stockpile . . . It's not supposed to be state stockpiles that they then use.

It's possible that what Kushner meant was that the states should use up their own resources before asking for material from the federal stockpile. But his pronouncements underscored an evident federal reluctance to wholeheartedly help the states.[36] During a well-publicized PPE shortage among emergency personnel, Trump suggested that some hospital medical workers were stealing masks for resale.[37] The point is that the federal government did not openly and transparently support state needs for PPE and ventilators, especially during early surges of COVID-19.

Governor Whitmer juggled multiple crises. She had to deflect resources from funds for water and education (earmarked to deprived areas of Michigan) toward disaster response. Her lockdown order was opposed in demonstrations by armed militia members who brought their long guns into the state capitol building while the legislature was in session. (Trump praised and encouraged them.) Two dams collapsed after decades-long neglect of upgrades, displacing residents and requiring emergency relief. The George Floyd protests brought initial looting in Detroit. In a conference call with other governors and President Trump, the president advised the governors "to dominate" their streets. Whitmer joined protesters in Detroit soon after, because she shared in their demand for racial justice, expressed in demonstrations throughout the United States.[38] Whitmer's leadership has been heroic, but she was put in a position of crisis management that is obviously unsustainable economically, as well as continually subject to Democratic–Republican governor–legislature politics.

Some of the militia members who occupied the Michigan capitol went on to be part of a plot by the "Wolverine Watchmen" to kidnap

Governor Whitmer and put her on "trial for treason." This conspiracy was surveilled by the FBI, and Whitmer was "moved around" for her safety. These details were made public after arrests of Wolverine Watchmen revealed misogynistic motivations and a goal to foment a civil war in the United States. Whitmer blamed the rhetoric of the Trump administration for inspiring this group. Right-wing extremism has been coalescing for decades in the United States, as well as world-wide.[39]

Conflicts between state governments and local officials have arisen when mayors and city managers have tried to address their immediate community needs with more restrictions than provided by state government. For example, states that reopened quickly, such as Florida, Georgia, and Arizona, have experienced COVID-19 surges, in the absence of state government mandates for masks and social distancing. Local mayors pressed advisories and official CDC guidelines to their populations, while at the same time pleading with their governors to issue more strict statewide edicts. Some of these same mayors and other local officials had earlier tried to resist state orders to reopen businesses, especially bars and restaurants, when COVID-19 cases were still on the rise. For a while, there was a trend to transfer mitigation decisions from state to local government.[40] However, as the progress of reopening clashed with surges in COVID-19 cases, this transfer of authority expired in some places.[41] Suffice it to say that intra-state tensions about how to manage COVID-19 response have been as complex and intense as state–federal government tensions.

Insufficient state funding has included budget cuts in disaster preparation materials and personnel. Crisis management on state levels during the COVID-19 pandemic has been the result of decades-long anti-government political activism and elective success. Motivations have included racism and refusal of collective responsibility for the conditions of poor and nonwhite Americans. The anti-government component of government has made government dysfunctional in normal life through routine budgetary cuts to social welfare and education programs, a process magnified by the pandemic. It is important to understand that the anti-government principles and values that have made the disaster more intense are playing out against preexisting erosion of physical and social infrastructure.

Positive and Negative Rights and the US Constitution

A general, international historical case can be made that pandemics legitimize government restrictions on normal freedoms.[42] However, in the United States, Republican, Conservative, and Libertarian political positions and expressions against pandemic mitigation, especially mask wearing and the closure of businesses, have called upon the Bill of Rights and general principles of individual liberty. The US constitutional perspective that government should stay out of private life and business rests on negative rights, or what the government is prohibited from doing. However, both public activism and normative legal theory can provide countervailing rights discourse. The George Floyd protests have been rights-based in a positive sense that contrasts with assertions of rights by protesters against quarantine, which rest on negative rights. In US constitutional terms, this positive–negative rights distinction, which is often attributed to Isaiah Berlin (1909–1997), amounts to the difference between what should not be done to citizens by government and what citizens demand from government in order to exercise their basic autonomy.

There are many ways government can make life worse for those governed by taking positive action, and President Ronald Reagan encapsulated fears of government interference with his "nine most terrifying words"—that is, "I'm from the government and I'm here to help." However, in complex societies where everyone does not know everyone else, there is great diversity of circumstances, and many projects can be financed and carried out for everyone, only from a powerful central authority. If help is needed, only the government can help. What may then become terrifying is government's unwillingness or inability to help. At that point, legal scholars and other theorists may begin to rethink the fundamental nature of rights in the US Constitution.

Ruthann Robson recently argued for "positive constitutionalism" in a pandemic, in contrast to the negative rights asserted by protesters against quarantine. Robson claims that we should have a "Constitution that is robust enough to recognize the rights of our people to have a government that puts our interests first and that actively and affirmatively protects our 'well-being.'"[43] Robson's argument translates rhetorical desires for top-down effective federal government care of the populace into constitutional interpretation. However, the mechanism for implementation, should such interpretation gain political traction, remains unclear. Would it require judicial review, new legislation, or a constitutional amendment? Such a shift would be sufficient to bring about more federal action if there were widespread expectations that the federal government be benevolent and responsible, rather than indifferent and lacking in disaster response and prevention obligations. Perhaps the positive-rights shift would be a formal version of the rhetoric of compassion. (Compassion will be considered in chapter 3 as part of a more extensive discussion of rhetoric during COVID-19.)

It is also unclear how negative rights or individual freedom from government interference can be applied in the current pandemic. If the COVID-19 virus were much less contagious, then individuals could meaningfully demand that they decide what risks they want to accept regarding their own health and life by congregating in large groups, not practicing social distancing, and not wearing masks. But contagion makes that kind of individual responsibility meaningless, because individuals cannot know whether others with whom they come in contact have been infected. Individuals cannot even know at any given time if they themselves have been infected—tests are valid only up to the time when the test is administered. This situation means that individuals have no knowledge about their own capacity to harm others. And the principle that we should not harm others is at least as venerable as any principle of individual rights that extends to movement, association, or expression (by showing one's face). Still, the principle of not harming others is not a constitutional principle, and apart from criminal law, which varies greatly among states, there is no general constitutional government obligation to protect citizens against one another.

There has been widespread complaint about the lack of federal leadership, specifically Trump's inability or unwillingness to unite the country in responding to COVID-19. However, such top-down unity could only effectively consist of general inspiring rhetoric and material and financial assistance to supplement state programs. To some extent, federal material and financial help have already been forthcoming, so that some of the frustration with the federal response has been a desire for a certain kind of rhetoric. There are no federal powers to do anything apart from supporting and supplying states. It is questionable whether the federal government could order quarantines and fairly certain that it has no power to order states to end quarantines or order people to return to work, apart from orders under the Defense Production Act that specific factories operate. Unifying rhetoric could frame general principles for local and specific interpretation and application. In reality, the structure of the US federal system, which can place certain kinds of on-the-ground official rule in the power of local officials, is a good match for this pandemic, because the virus crops up in different ways and at different times, throughout the states. However, this is not to say that local versus state conflict can be smoothly resolved in any particular case. And it fails to take into account the fact that state borders are permeable.

To sum up: Federal response powers in a public health disaster such as COVID-19 are limited without extraordinary measures, which were not taken by November 2020. Response powers and authority reside in the states, with support from the federal government, which in this case has not been as robust as demanded. The states have shown willingness to assert their constitutional and statutory (Stafford Act) rights against the federal government. Within states, disaster response has been contentious when Democratic governors have been opposed by Republican legislatures and more local Conservatives and Libertarians. Also, Republican state governments have been opposed by urban mayors requiring stricter mitigation. Some individuals, in resisting pandemic mitigation measures, have relied on the idea of their constitutional rights against government interference, but the validity of such rights is arguable in light of the international history of governments in pandemics, a positive-right interpretation of the Constitution, and the irrelevance of negative rights to situations of contagion that evokes the principle that we should not harm one another.

But there is instantaneous as well as traditional politics, or activism as well as official political action. Just as COVID-19 has been politicized in addition to the problems caused by the disease itself, so have the George Floyd/Black Lives Matter protests, which can be understood as a grassroots demand for positive rights. In Portland, Oregon, both peaceful and violent protests had been taking place on the streets for one hundred days by the end of August 2020. The federal government interceded at one point, with troops without badges in unmarked vehicles. Several protesters were taken off the streets and put into unmarked vehicles without apparent grounds for arrest. This intervention was apparently directly ordered by President Trump, who blamed Antifa followers and the Democratic mayor for civic unrest. In late August, a Trump supporter who was part of a six-hundred-car anti-protest caravan was shot and killed, and a suspect who proclaimed Antifa affiliation was shot and killed by police during his arrest.[44] But the history of race relations in Portland, which has included legally enforced segregation, as well as Oregon laws prohibiting black people from entering the state or buying property, raises the question of whether there is broad and deep support for the protests sparked by George Floyd's killing. In recent years, gentrification has driven black residents out of the same poor neighborhoods they were historically restricted to. The irony of having "Black Lives Matter" signs in these areas has not gone unnoticed, and this has led some to claim that the Portland protests are politically opportunistic, as well as expressive of outrage against racial injustice.[45] This does not vitiate reasons for outrage, although it suggests that all levels of politics, including activism, are complicated.

3

RHETORIC AND THE US CULTURE WARS

"When Dorothy, the Tin Man, the Cowardly Lion, and the Scarecrow all find the Wizard, they hear a loud voice booming all around them, telling them to come back another time. It almost sounds as if the Wizard of Oz is some kind of god, sending his message down from the clouds.

"But then Toto, Dorothy's dog, discovers that the Wizard is no god. In fact, he's just a guy operating a bunch of controls behind a green curtain. When Toto rips the curtain to the side, the Wizard of Oz realizes he's been found out, and tries to cover it up by shouting over his loudspeaker, 'Pay no attention to that man behind the curtain!'"

—*The Wizard of Oz* [1]

At The Villages, a retirement community in Northern Florida, some of the residents organized a parade in support of President Trump. They draped "Make America Great Again" banners and US flags on their golf carts and drove around in their compound. The parade became contentious when counter-demonstrators emerged. On June 28, 2020, Trump retweeted a video in which an elderly white man in the golf-cart parade pumps his fist in the air, calling out "White Power," and his call is echoed by another white man standing nearby. Trump's retweet was immediately met with accusations that Trump was endorsing White Supremacy and sowing division at a time when everyone in the United States was struggling with COVID-19, together with recent George Floyd–protest awareness of the extent and historical depth of white anti-black racism. Trump's retweet was taken down in three hours, and the next day his press secretary said that he had not heard the White Power callout and was merely thanking his supporters.[2] By the time of this incident, Trump's history of racist remarks, slurs against people of color, and apparent welcome of White Supremacist supporters was already well known among Democrats and other critics.

Trump's insensitivity to racism, or his approval of racism as a political motive that benefits him, or even his appetite for taunting nonwhite people and white liberals, or his racism, is the subject of the golf-cart White Power account and many other similar accounts. Here, I would like to consider the form of the golf-cart white power incident, how it came to human attention, and the kind of thing it is.

The entire golf-cart white power incident was a matter of rhetoric. The golf-cart parade was a rhetorical gesture, as was resistance from protesters; Trump's retweet was rhetorical speech; Twitter itself is a rhetorical tool; and Trump's removal of the retweet was a rhetorical move that showed his flexibility in rhetorical discourse—abrupt changes in course are rhetorical flourishes, like feints in fencing. Trump may be generally ignorant and lacking in moral principles. He uses the presidency like an egoist with tunnel vision. But Trump is a master rhetorician.

It is important to understand what rhetoric is and is not, at this time, in order to understand Trump's presidency and the historical period we have been living through. However, the subject of rhetoric can connect distinct topics in surprising ways, and the best way to get a handle on this subject is not obvious. Here, I approach rhetoric through compassion and its absence in Trump's role in the US culture wars. The rhetorical nature of these wars suggests that Trump is this nation's first President of Rhetoric. The heart of this chapter is a discussion of the George Floyd protests, which express compassion and are rhetorical in demanding police reform. Police reform and the institutional changes demanded along with it involve positive rights. In the twentieth century, the nature of positive rights, as motivated by compassion, was introduced by the 1948 Universal Declaration of Human Rights. The chapter ends with a recent example of how even rigid constitutional rhetoric can shift from negative to positive rights, given help from a quintessentially American fictional character.

COMPASSION AND ITS LACK

The intense crisis of COVID-19 has both laid bare preexisting inequalities and brought forth extraordinary attitudes of compassion. Compassion motivated the initial mitigation projects of quarantine and social distancing, which had the explicit aim of protecting the elderly when they were believed to be the only ones vulnerable to the virus. The implicit aim was to prevent overwhelming the health-care system with large numbers of COVID-19 patients at the same time. Health care itself has been recast from a corporate enterprise to an industry of compassion. The public has repeatedly expressed gratitude and compassion for overworked doctors and nurses, capped by evening ceremonies of acclaim and celebrations of their heroism in heavily burdened areas. Furthermore, compassion has been evident when police and other officials have expressed common cause with antiracist protesters after George Floyd's murder.

Indeed, compassion seems to have been the overwhelming motivation after so many witnessed the obscene injustice of George Floyd's last minutes. The public display of such compassion has been expressive, evocative, moral, and rhetorical. It is expressive because people can show (demonstrate) what they are thinking and feeling. Our recognition of compassion in others strengthens our own compassion, and that is how the protests and demonstrations have been evocative. The sharing of compassion for victims of injustice and displays of commitment to correcting that injustice are forms of moral action. Compassion is a feeling, and as such its public display is a form of rhetoric. As just noted, the George Floyd protests are not merely rhetorical, but in this chapter, the focus is on their rhetorical aspect and political rhetoric more broadly. Rhetoric is powerful but seldom recognized for what it is. The feeling and emotional components of rhetoric easily preempt both the cognitive aspects of rhetoric and the reasoning and facts external to rhetoric. Contemporary neuroscience supports the idea that human beings are hard-wired to respond faster and more intensely to information that is processed in the parts of the brain that process feelings and emotions than in the parts that process thoughts and reasoning.[3]

The feelings and expressions of compassion for the elderly, health-care workers, and George Floyd are politically bipartisan. President Trump's call for the military to "dominate" American streets struck many as undemocratic, also in a bipartisan way. His call was met with widespread outrage, on the grounds that it was unconstitutional, divisive, and tone-deaf, as well as lacking in compassion.[4] Soon after that, the president implied that George Floyd in heaven was looking down on him with approval for an uptick in employment figures when unemployment decreased from 16 percent to 13 percent! Those who had been appalled by Trump's apparent ongoing lack of compassion were shocked by his attempt to appropriate the subject of the protests for his own political purposes.[5] And at that point, the presidential politics was obviously both partisan and self-serving. Trump's attempt to further his reelection was obvious, given that he had touted the powerful pre-COVID-19 economy as his distinctive and unique accomplishment in office.

THE RHETORICAL NATURE OF THE US CULTURE WARS

Overall, including public compassion, presidential partisanship, and Democratic opposition, there is a strong rhetorical aspect to the early twenty-first-century US culture wars, which is often overlooked as rhetoric, because people go straight to the content. The term *rhetoric*, here, refers to public speech, gesture, and performance that are all somewhat self-contained. Much of life on-screen in social media is also rhetorical in this sense, as is much of Donald Trump's presidency, and as may be the George Floyd protests. The oppositional or dialectical nature of US federalism is echoed in strong cultural differences throughout the United States, which render disaster preparation, mitigation, and response, always local. This local aspect of COVID-19 means that national unity in the present disaster would mainly be rhetorical. The failure to understand how, if we had it during COVID-19, national unity would be mainly rhetorical leads to much frustration and anguish—and more rhetoric, which, like the idealized rhetoric of unity, does not identify itself as rhetoric.

After the 2016 presidential campaign, pundits liked to say that Trump's supporters took him seriously but not literally, while his progressive opponents and critics took him literally but not seriously.[6] Soon into his presidency, his opponents and critics took him both literally and seriously, and his supporters continued to take him seriously, but maybe even less literally. They understood that he did not reason linearly or logically, on the basis of factually true premises, and this was acceptable to them. Trump's rhetoric has been extremely successful, as evident in the vast number of those who voted for him in the 2020 election. Political speech is rhetorical, but voting is action in reality. We don't know whether those who voted for Trump were motivated by his rhetoric or by other unspoken reasons (such as, for instance, simple fear of change).

THE NATION'S FIRST RHETORICAL PRESIDENT

Left out by the dichotomy of seriously–literally is, exactly, this idea of rhetoric. President Trump will likely be the nation's first rhetorical president. He puts on a show in which truth, civility, consistency, and even competence appear, to him and his "base," to be unnecessary for fulfilling his role as president. All that matters is his discourse or the "narrative" he constructs. The federal structure discussed in chapter 2 reinforces the rhetorical aspect of Trump's role in disaster. Trump does not have the legal federal power to practically unite the United States concerning this disaster without taking extraordinary measures, such as a Declaration of Major Disaster according to 401(a) of the Stafford Act or comprehensively invoking the Defense Production Act. But he has repeatedly spurned opportunities to accept COVID-19 as a major national disaster, and his rhetorical efforts have been dedicated to downplaying the effects of COVID-19 and implying that it is unpatriotic or destructive to national unity to view COVID-19 as a major national disaster. For example, when a reporter asked him what he had to say to Americans who were scared (on a day when 200 were dead and 14,000 ill from the virus), he replied:

> I say you're a terrible reporter, that's what I say. I think it's a very nasty question, and I think it's a very bad signal that you're putting out to the American people.[7]

Trump has consistently responded to COVID-19 in rhetorical terms, claiming, for instance, that increasing the number of tests merely increases the official reported number of cases, as though there were no underlying reality to be reported.[8] This oblivion concerning underlying reality, or what most would simply call "reality," suggests that Trump not only is the first rhetorical president but also may believe that being the President of the United States means that he is the President of the Rhetoric of the United States, and nothing further. If he did believe that, it would explain much of his aggression toward news reporters. Reporters believe and present their work as though they are talking about things outside of their reports, while for Trump, there may not be anything outside of such reports. And not coincidentally, it would also explain his many lies—if there is no reality apart from what one says, especially what the President of Rhetoric says, then there is no such thing as a lie![9]

Of course, Trump does act, as in signing the Coronavirus, Aid, Relief, and Economic Security (CARES) Act passed by Congress and withdrawing from the World Health Organization because of their slowness in recognizing COVID-19 as a global pandemic and their favoritism toward China despite its meager contribution to the WHO budget compared to the United States. But he then recasts such actions in rhetoric, such as requesting that his name appear on CARES Act stimulus checks sent to the American people, and casting the WHO as complicit in China's downplaying of the then-epidemic, while implying that the SARS-CoV-2 virus originated in a Chinese laboratory. The result is that his stated reasons and motivations for such actions lack credibility for those who are not generally within his rhetorical bubble.[10]

Many of Trump's actions have exceeded rhetoric in sinister ways—brutal immigration policies and retaliation against whistle-blowers. But he somehow gets away with this, perhaps because rhetoric is his epistemological home base. If he can describe an otherwise unjustified or inexcusable action within his rhetorical bubble, without alienating his supporters, then that is what he counts as success. And it is success if those who agree with his rhetoric vote for him and those he endorses win and in turn support him, because he controls the votes of his base. In other words, politically, rhetoric functions as propaganda, and its political use is to motivate people to take political action that benefits the rhetorician. But on its own terms, the promise of rhetoric such as Trump's is that a story will continually be told which is internally coherent and independent of reality, but enough of a facsimile of reality to take the place of factually descriptive discourse. The truth becomes "bent" to fit a falsely optimistic narrative of American greatness in which Trump and his supporters, united by their real biases, are the heroes.

Trump's ability to spin out this story, while a pandemic and new awareness of racial injustice traumatize the nation, is very creative. The bad news is that it is not effective or constructive governance; the good news is that Trump's "genius" is probably unique—that is, it won't happen again. The news we don't have yet is whether the extravagance of having Trump as president, with both his supporters and his critics taking him seriously, is something we can afford. If it turns out we can afford it, then, in reality, the United States will emerge as a far more sophisticated society than its traditional persona of innocence could have ever suggested. If we cannot afford its stress on democratic institutions and collective individual values and stamina, as well as material wealth, well, in that case, Trump will have broken the bank.

Presuming that only discourse is relevant to truth and that what people believe determines what is true is a metaphysical doctrine. When it is agreed that beliefs ought to be tested by findings from history, journalism, and science, which occur external to them, this kind of metaphysics is replaced by realism. The US culture wars are not at this time solely matters of incompatible bubbles or values but also incompatible views about how truth is to be determined—by consistency with pre-accepted self-contained rhetoric or by reference to information external to that rhetoric. But again, this is a matter of the content of what people believe and their assumptions in believing it. If those who create the rhetoric of Trump and the rhetoric of conspiracy theories (see chapters 8 and 9) know that they are entertaining and manipulating their audiences with fictional accounts or lies, then the epistemological and metaphysical distinctions fall away and only moral ones remain— that is, should one tell the truth, or are fiction and lies permissible?

There are also psychological issues pertaining to lying. In *Too Much and Never Enough: How My Family Created the World's Most Dangerous Man*, Mary L. Trump, President Donald J. Trump's tell-all niece, simply assumes that the psychological pathology of the president is important enough to destroy the United States (and with that, presumably, the world). She writes in her prologue:

But now the stakes are far higher than they've ever been before; they are literally life and death. Unlike any previous time in his life, Donald's failings cannot be hidden or ignored because they threaten us all. . . . Donald, following the lead of my grandfather and with the complicity, silence, and inaction of his siblings, destroyed my father. I can't let him destroy my country.[11]

Trump's apparent aspiration to "kingship" is important, not only because the founders of the Constitution sought to avoid monarchy in the structure of US government but also because it is so personal. Trump's psychological pathology manifests as delusions of grandeur, because the United States is not a monarchy. But juxtaposed against the American aversion to despotism is the enduring popularity of the British royals. The structure of the British monarchy, in reality as well as metaphorically, has a history of the expansion of a personal household. To begin with, the British monarchy is officially described as supported by the Royal Household of the United Kingdom. The Royal Household assists the queen as head of state, organizes public ceremonies, and preserves the royal collection. As in the history of other Western European monarchies, posts originally held by the monarch's domestic servants developed into major administrative positions. For example, the Lord Chancellor began as head of the monarch's writing office but became keeper of the Great Seal and the main officer of state. Similar ascensions developed for the Lord Steward and the Master of the Horse; the Keeper of the Privy Purse remains personal treasurer to the sovereign and also oversees charitable donations and grants.[12]

More theoretically, the personal domestic origins of modern monarchies live on through metaphors still used in the modern state, which disguise great impersonal authority and power[13]—for example, "the Home Office" in the United Kingdom or "the Department of Homeland Security" in the United States. In this sense, the presentation of government through metaphors of home or domesticity is an important propaganda tool. The whole nation can be reconfigured as a collective home. The Department of Homeland Security was formed after 9/11, along with new repressive and undemocratic measures that eventually included unauthorized surveillance, searches, and torture during the "War on Terror."[14]

The literal personal origins of the British monarchy continue to be evident beyond the nomenclature of high office. The British royals continually supply the news with drama, not for political reasons or as the result of social controversies arising from their charitable causes, but for their endless personal upheavals involving marital infidelity, sexual misconduct, hurt feelings, and, of course, fashion. All of these soap opera–worthy exploits revolve around their "private" lives. Indeed, Buckingham Palace is proactive as well as reactive to various leaks of the latest gossip. [15]

The brilliance of this production lies in the immense popularity of the reserved and dignified persona that Queen Elizabeth II has been able to maintain since her coronation in 1953. President Trump admires the queen and has reported an "amazing chemistry" with her. [16] But even though Roseanne Barr has dubbed him the nation's "first woman president" (for his display of negative female stereotypical behavior), [17] Trump does not have royal gravitas. Nevertheless, presidential rhetoric metastasizes: If people don't believe his niece, her book only adds to the obsession with his personality; if people do believe his niece, the same thing happens (insofar as there is no political appetite for invoking the Twenty-fifth Amendment). [18]

This suggests that the new disorder in the American president's administration is related not only to a shift from descriptive discourse into rhetoric but also to considerable change in the content of both discourse and rhetoric about government. The main content of administration discourse, both from and about the administration, used to be about national security, the economy, the common good, taxation, and other collective subjects. But during the Trump administration, it has focused on the whims, rudeness, and character flaws of the president, which are all aspects of personality.

The substitution of personality for professionalism enables dangerous behavior that administrative actions based on rules would preclude. After President Trump contracted COVID-19 (presumptively at a "super-spreader" event in the Rose Garden on September 26, 2020[19]), he apparently declined to follow medical advice to quarantine. He related his decision process in a video released from Walter Reed Hospital on October 3, 2020:

> I had no choice because I just didn't want to stay in the White House. I was given that alternative: stay in the White House, lock yourself in, don't ever leave, don't even go to the Oval Office, just stay upstairs and enjoy it. Don't see people, don't talk to people, and

just be done with it and I can't do that, I had to be out front and this is America, this is the United States, the greatest country in the world. This is the most powerful country in the world. I can't be locked up in a room upstairs and totally safe and just say "Hey, whatever happens, happens." I can't do that.[20]

Adherence to official medical directives from the CDC would have obligated Trump to quarantine instead of continuing with activities that could and probably did result in contagion among top Republican leadership, including himself. A more conscientious person than Trump would have quarantined when advised to do so. However, the issue here is not the quality or morality of Trump's personality, but rather how he performed his official duties as actions stemming from himself, personally, instead of from professional obligations. While no law was broken, a prior administrative directive to follow CDC recommendations would have resulted in presidential quarantine and avoidance of contagion before then. Professionalism would have required a president to follow such CDC directives from his own administration. Government by and through office holders' personalities is not professionalism. While Trump's presidency has been attractive to his followers because he is not a professional politician, the position of president is a professional position. If amateurs are employed in professional positions, their prior amateur status does not thereby exempt them from the professional obligations of their new roles.

The political genre of intimate personality was also present in Joe Biden's presidential candidacy. Biden had related personal issues in his writing, during the Democratic National Convention, and in subsequent interviews, debates, and speeches, including a response to a Trump scandal about disrespect for slain members of the military. He continually evoked the loss of his son, Beau, who died from brain cancer at the age of forty-six. During interviews, Biden produced his son's rosary that he carries with him all the time.[21] The question is not the quality of the content of such extremely personal disclosure but whether it is relevant to governing. There is no doubt that voters eagerly peruse and discuss personal information about elected officials.

A presidency of rhetorical personality combined with both party-driven and marginal (e.g., conspiracy-driven) politics has been a disaster within the disaster of COVID-19. But what if the presidential personality is emotional or nonprofessional in ways that line up with virtues? At the Democratic National Convention on August 21, 2020, Joe Biden gave a nomination acceptance speech that was aspirational in calling for hope and emotional in expressing compassion, and he continued these themes into his victory speech. Throughout the virtual convention, presentations from ordinary Americans and political supporters emphasized Joe Biden's compassion and empathy. Issues and plans are on display on his website, but the ultimate appeal was based on Biden's character, with strong emphasis on how he overcame personal tragedy with the loss of his first wife and one daughter and then his adult son, Beau.[22] We know that this kind of personal campaigning works. Still, insofar as the work of governing is a matter of plans that are implemented to address problems, it does not go beyond political rhetoric.

Rhetoric can disguise itself as sincere expression, based on how politicians conceive of their audience. American racism is layered in the political sphere. Donald Trump has spoken of people of color in disparaging terms—for instance, in reference to "shithole countries," constant disparagement of women of color in politics, and criminalization of immigrants from Mexico and Central America, as well as black Americans. This discourse, combined with insinuations that multifamily dwellings in the suburbs will increase crime because people of color will be their inhabitants, have led Democratic and other critics to insist that Trump is a racist. By this they mean that in his heart and mind, he believes his implications of nonwhite inferiority and criminality. However, the situation is more complicated than the question of whether Trump or anyone else who says such things is a racist. A politician's motives for saying anything unrelated to the work of governing can be a desire to manipulate voters.[23]

In *Rage*, Bob Woodward reports (with accompanied recordings) seventeen on-the-record interviews with President Trump, beginning in February 2020. In those interviews, Trump revealed knowledge about the danger of COVID-19, which his public dismissals of the pandemic contradicted. And he also both dismissed the idea of an obligation to examine his own white racial privilege and acknowledged that racism was deeply embedded in American life. While critics have seized on the fact of lies and apparent ignorance of white privilege as evidence of Trump's bad character, of equal interest is Trump's revelation that he has said things that he doesn't himself believe, presumably because supporters and potential voters want to believe them. This was not a simple matter of saying what was known to be untrue but living it on public display. While the president was in his words "downplaying" the pandemic, he was seen playing golf, conducting rallies, and traveling freely without mask wearing by himself or his associates and followers. This occurred after he had remarked on the airborne nature of SARS-CoV-2. Here, political rhetoric goes beyond mere speech to include not only gestures but also full-fledged acting—Trump played the role of a president who did not believe that COVID-19 was a serious threat to health and life.

If we focus on Trump's mendacity and racism in personal senses, we may miss how political craft has been revealed through the Woodward interviews. The manipulation of members of the electorate who are already racist or gullible about a pandemic is a form of propaganda that, unlike traditional distortions of the truth, does not require convincing anybody of anything. It is enough if people are already racist or misinformed or are known to subscribe to conspiracy theories. Such identifiable beliefs can then be "hailed" in a political context to create electoral loyalty. The more bizarre such beliefs are, the easier it is to manipulate those who hold them, because recognition from an authority figure will validate them, after they have been hailed by mention of what they believe. The more disparaged the bizarre beliefs are by members of educated communities, the stronger will be the affinity and loyalty to the authority figure who also pretends to hold these bizarre beliefs. It's easy to criticize racist or scientifically ignorant beliefs that are used as bait in this way. But should more attractive professions of good character, compassion, and noble values get a pass?

It is ironic that there is bipartisan agreement, with no apparent censorship, concerning a number of facts about COVID-19, despite President Trump's optimistic rhetoric about conquering the invisible enemy. Such facts include numbers of positive cases according to testing and reported deaths; effectiveness of different treatments and preventions, such as wearing masks; unemployment figures and claims; GNP data; housing statistics; and financial market data and reports. All of this information is circulated by numerous government, media, and institutional outlets. Trump's initial attempt to deal with COVID-19 treatment rhetorically by promoting the malaria drug hydroxychloroquine failed after a statistical review showed the drug to be ineffective or harmful to hospitalized patients with the virus. [24]

But people love rhetoric, so a fact here or there is unlikely to punc-
ture a major bubble. Nor does an internal contradiction matter much.
For instance, despite Trump's regular downplaying of COVID-19, the
requirement that attendees sign waivers of liability for contracting
COVID-19 apparently did not deter some thousands of Trump supporters from buying advance tickets for a Trump campaign rally on July 20,
2020, in Tulsa, Oklahoma.[25] However, hundreds of thousands of tickets
were purchased through TikTok by teenagers who had no intention of
attending, which raised initial expectations within the Trump reelection
campaign that one million people would attend the Tulsa rally.[26] In
reality, only about 6,200 attended an arena that could hold 19,000, and
an overflow building was never used. An outdoor presidential speech
was canceled due to scant attendance and the stage dismantled.[27] But
the low attendance and reports that masks and social distancing were
not required did not deter Trump from planning other scheduled campaign events. In other words, the rhetoric surrounding Trump coexists
with sober practical reports about the pandemic, as well as reports
about events featuring that rhetoric.

Trump performs rhetorically on the Right/Red branch of the contemporary political spectrum, which is taken literally by his critics and
others aghast at his antics, but it has been rare for Trump's opponents
to formulate rhetorical responses. Many have mocked and made fun of
him, but comedy is not the same as rhetoric. Rhetoric is serious, not-
literal, and it occurs on a level of communication that is self-sustaining
and self-contained. Rhetoric feeds on itself and does not need external
references—that is, facts—to validate it. Comedy, by contrast, mainly
works because it is not self-contained but depends on reinterpretations
of what it refers to outside of its discourse. Rhetoric cannot be effectively opposed with comedy, including satire and ridicule. Rather, rhetoric can be effectively opposed only by stronger rhetoric. And so, finally, there was a turning point.

THE GEORGE FLOYD PROTESTS

As noted in chapter 2, President Trump ordered National Guard troops
to occupy Washington, DC, on the day after his Bible-thumping trip
across Lafayette Square to St. John's Church. Mayor Muriel E. Bowser

of Washington, DC, then ordered the words "Black Lives Matter" painted in giant yellow letters from curb to curb along a street leading to the White House. And it was at that time that Mayor Bowser requested that the National Guard troops ordered by Trump be removed from her city jurisdiction. Trump removed them two days later.[28]

Those giant yellow letters were a rhetorical response to Trump's rhetoric about the "violent Antifa" demonstrators whom he had cleared from Lafayette Square. The giant yellow letters not only shouted back at his race baiting but also raised the rhetorical stakes of that particular confrontation by evoking the yellow brick road in *The Wizard of Oz*, which leads to a scary tyrant with no real substance apart from the ability to broadcast propaganda. This is something that many Americans understand in ways that bypass cognition—Mayor Bowser created a relevant, mocking, rhetorical response to Trump's rhetoric at that time. Her response, of course, occurred within the bigger and longer context of the George Floyd protests.

The George Floyd mass protests have appeared to be more substantial than rhetorical in content, but they may in historical retrospect turn out to be mainly rhetorical, albeit spectacularly so. Moreover, the rhetoric about the protests, which is rhetoric about rhetoric, consisting of speech in the public auditorium (e.g., punditry on television, social media, and the press) began with intellectual sophistication. In addition to discussion of the injustice of George Floyd's murder and wider recounting of other young black male homicide victims of police officers, the disproportionate number of blacks in prison and ongoing poverty of, and racism against, African Americans has been discussed historically as a legacy of lynching and Jim Crow as well as slavery. Also, the disproportionate number of black COVID-19 infections and deaths due to preexisting medical conditions, as well as low-wage service jobs with high human contact and the ongoing stress caused by both violence and microaggression, have been related to the US history of oppression and discrimination.[29] This situation in turn has led to discussion of a need for structural change in employment, education, and health care. Such deeper-than-usual awareness in public discussion of issues that were previously confined to scholarly work would likely not have occurred without the spectacle of mass protests and their calls for change. The spectacle could then be interpreted as objection to systemic racism, as an unjust structure needing change.

The powerfully rhetorical George Floyd protests are now a fulcrum for change. But no matter what changes do or do not follow, those who participated in the protests will be able to show pictures and videos of themselves and the crowds they were part of, for years to come. This is meaningful to individuals. In addition to its contribution to individual biography, it will indelibly be part of collective American history. But so far, these protests are little more than rhetorical or expressive—that is, self-contained. Real change occurs over time, throughout daily life, thought, and institutional practices, and we need to wait to see whether that has happened.

The George Floyd protests fulfill Marx's dream of liberated workers having the time for civic engagement. All apparent races, with a white majority, were apparent during the first months of the protests, and members of all socioeconomic classes (especially the generic middle class) were present. Without furloughs, terminations, and the freedom to work at home, together with economic respite from the CARES Act, including stimulus checks, unemployment compensation, and moratoria on rent and mortgage payments, that many people would not have had the time to fill the streets on weekdays and weeknights.[30] The worthy causes of outrage and calls for police reform, as well as overall indignation about long-standing anti-black racism(s), seemed to justify the risk of contracting and spreading COVID-19 in crowds that did not allow for much social distance. A lot of people seized the opportunity to let off a lot of steam, and the immediate economic circumstances of many of them, if not their long-term economic prospects, made it possible for them to do that. It is unknown what will happen when the mass public presence abates, as people go back to work and colleges reopen. If more restaurants, bars, and public recreation venues were permanently reopened, would the same crowds remember George Floyd, or would new crowds be able to take their place to protest new and different injustices?

We should also note the commonality of George Floyd's inability to breathe and the serious effects of COVID-19 as an illness. (Added to that is the coincidence that Floyd had survived COVID-19, before his death in Minneapolis.[31]) However, no speculation as to cause can take away the evident sincerity of protesters. George Floyd's death was directly witnessed by a global audience. Social psychologist Paul Slovic has shown that people are not moved by hearing about large numbers of injuries and death, but rather by single cases.[32] The singleness of George Floyd's death over the span of eight minutes was subsequently seen by the millions (billions?) of viewers in the global audience. That intimate connection, shortly after the event, moved them. The emotional responses to these viewings would have been immediate, with cognitive analyses and calls for structural reform to come later.

The George Floyd protests hold out prospects of radical police reform and hope for broader racial justice in society. These protests against the murder of George Floyd have the historical potential of real participatory democracy, to the extent that those with power and authority meant it, as they spoke of a need for police reform and/or structural change everywhere in the United States. If such reform and change occur, it could be national reform, evoked by local responses. This would show us that US federalism allows for bottom-up change, in our time. There could be national change if there is official federal top-down change, similar to the legislation of the 1960s civil rights movement. But there could also be national change if there are reforms within police departments, because although police departments are local, if they all reform, it would add up to national change.

Until the fulcrum of the protests seemed to begin to change the world, the intransigence of US police aggression against people of color was a major component of the culture wars. First there was "Blue Lives Matter," in response to "Black Lives Matter," either creating a false dichotomy between the lives of white police officers and black people or falsely implying that "Black Lives Matter" was intended to mean that only black lives matter. This was followed by George Floyd protest presidential rhetoric of "When the looting starts, the shooting starts."[33] In addition, there has been rhetorical blame in the president's claim that the antifascist group Antifa was responsible for looting and violence during protests. At the same time, there has been an increase in more sober official concern about the White Supremacist Boogaloo Movement's white right-wing extremist presence in protests—the movement's aim is to start a second US Civil War.[34] Physical violence breaks the bubble of rhetoric, although whether it leads to real-life change in a historical sense generally depends on whether it is politically effective or merely criminal.

In any case, the size of protests in the midst of the COVID-19 pandemic feeds on itself, as does fame, especially in an age of instant imagery. Many are famous simply because they are famous, and big crowds can grow bigger because they are already very big—and famous. The protest fame is instant, because the protests become reality television as they occur. It remains to be seen whether there will be enough who return to work and school to make such large protests impractical, or if continuing unemployment will result in poverty so dire that there is not enough energy to protest, or whether further relief for such poverty will continue to create more leisure for political participation, or if resurgence of COVID-19 will sicken too many for continued focus on protesting. Or?

We do not know whether protests have to occur continually in order to motivate and sustain change. We do know that the George Floyd protests by the third week resulted in the beginning of processes of police reform in at least two states. In Minnesota, city and state efforts to defund police were put into political motion.[35] The New York State legislature more promptly passed legislation banning chokeholds and requiring police departments throughout the state to begin meetings with their communities over the next nine months.[36] We do not know how effectively, and for how long, such reforms will be implemented— that is, whether they will become an abiding part of police and community culture.

COMPASSION AND POSITIVE RIGHTS

Academic exhortation and normative legal theory also contribute to the George Floyd protests by constructing aspirational schema or conceptual frameworks. These more formal expressions may share the motivation of compassion. Compassion can be an infectious concern for those worse off than oneself. Compassion is a generalized concern for another, including recognition of their situation and some degree of respect. It does not guarantee a feeling or belief that the object of compassion is an equal, although it is more spontaneous than pity, which can be a dutiful response. Compassion involves a change within the compassionate person, whereas pity can leave the one pitying as they were.

Empathy goes a step beyond compassion, in requiring an ability to imagine oneself in the situation of another. Empathy is thus closer to the recognition of equality than compassion. Any authorized change in constitutionalism from negative to positive rights, as discussed in chapter 2, would likely be initiated by those who did not need recognition of such positive rights, because those who do need them do not have the political and social power to change how the US Constitution is interpreted. Moreover, it is the better-off who have the leisure to envision improved societal circumstances for those oppressed and disadvantaged. This is why so many observers were encouraged by the large presence of white people in the George Floyd protests.[37]

The white protesters who swelled the crowds and the institutional declarations in white-dominated organizations that followed—the myriad "George Floyd statements"—were likely motivated by compassion, although once the trend was under way, the desire to visibly conform to respectable progressive norms would have been another motivation. Compassion is better than pity in terms of equality, but it lacks the identification with its objects that empathy requires. And, of course, empathy thereby ranks higher on the scale of altruistic virtues. Empathy also has the potential to become a political motivation, as I will soon suggest.

Those who signed the George Floyd statements and made other pronouncements, as well as white protesters who became newly aware of US anti-black racism, were unlikely to have experienced empathy, because of the newness of their awareness.[38] The problem with compassion in a situation like this is that the lack of an experience of equality with those who are oppressed keeps demands for change in an emotional rhetorical space. To enter an egalitarian and thereby potentially political rhetorical space, empathetic identification with the victims of racism would be necessary. Empathy for victims of injustice means that empathizers share their sense of injustice. Given the antidiscrimination legislation of the civil rights movement, perceived racial injustice is not only moral but already political. It is not political in the sense of allegiance to a party, but political because it already has a legal foundation.

The political response to the George Floyd protests begins with legislation regarding police reform, and, as noted, the protests have indeed inspired efforts toward that end. (Police reform will be discussed in chapter 5.) But to underscore the general rhetorical nature of the protests themselves, it may help to realize that even though such protests have been risky in a pandemic, and more immediately risky when police response has been brutal, as protests, they do not require commitment beyond a willingness to physically participate. One can physically participate in a protest without making further commitments to working on the mechanics for change, overseeing the efficacy of such change, or voting for candidates who promise such change and then holding them accountable. The real question in terms of social and political justice is how white-dominant organizations throughout society, as well as white individuals, will change their actions. A statement in and of itself may be compassionate, but beyond that, without action, it will prove at best aspirational and at worst superficial and hypocritical.

Nevertheless, aspiration is important. The premier global organization for world peace and general humanitarianism, the United Nations, has been rhetorically aspirational since it was founded in 1945. There is no international government to enforce its declarations of human rights and no mechanism to prevent even member nations from violating them. In anticipation of the UN's 1948 Universal Declaration of Human Rights (UDHR), Jacques Maritain, in his 1947 "Grounds for an International Declaration of Human Rights," referred to the British Bill of Rights and the American Bill of Rights, as well as the French Declaration of the Rights of Man and Citizen, as foundational for UDHR. The reliance on these declarations drew from their doctrines of negative rights, or rights based on what is impermissible for governments to do to citizens. Maritain claimed that these rights had already been incorporated into modern founding documents by the time the United Nations had been formed. The new purpose of UDHR was to add doctrines of positive rights for all humankind. [39] Articles 22–29 describe these as rights to social security, desirable work and joining trade unions, rest and leisure, adequate living standards, education, participation in the cultural life of the community, a social order articulating UDHR, and freedom from state or personal interference in the rights set forth in UDHR.

Not only are the positive rights declared by the United Nations aspirational, but it is also not clear how they can be claimed to be universal, insofar as not all nations have endorsed them, and there is no apparatus for correcting or punishing nations that violate them internally. There is a further limitation on the notion of universal rights in that the United Nations has found it necessary to constantly reiterate the rights of minorities, women, children, and other vulnerable groups, through hundreds of declarations since its founding. All of these declarations are inclusive in their language and morally good, but they have no more force or mechanisms for enforcement than UDHR.[40] Moreover, the specific declarations seem to be redundant, because if all humans have rights, then so do women, children, indigenous people, disabled people, elderly people, refugees, members of racial, religious, and ethnic minority groups, and others for whom the United Nations has claimed human rights. Nevertheless, as aspiration for the entire world, the ongoing iterations of human rights are an important part of the UN's world rhetorical role.

Although rhetoric, or any type or instance of rhetoric as belonging to a type, is self-contained, creating rhetoric is a real-world activity outside of rhetoric. The production of rhetoric in all of its forms is a real-life practice, a series of activities—such as making speeches, demonstrating or protesting, or even composing rules or norms for the creation of rhetoric. It is therefore not surprising that the UN has a robust answer to the question "How is the UN responding to COVID-19?" The UN is responding with a series of humanitarian declarations, as well as a relief fund. The secretary-general issued a comprehensive response on June 25, 2020, calling for a global effort budgeted at $7 billion, of which less than $2 billion had been raised.[41] While a global response to COVID-19 is unlikely to materialize at this time, it may be important to have that as an ideal, an aspiration, against which to criticize ineffective or obstructive responses by national governments and factions within them.

Also, we can still learn from UDHR's inclusion of positive rights, especially a positive right to protection by the government. As discussed in chapter 2, the US constitutional tradition has focused on rights that protect citizens from government. Resistance against lockdowns and mask-wearing edicts has drawn on that tradition, in some cases against state governments. But widespread vulnerability due to a new disease might make some people, as informed by experts, more receptive to the positive right of protection by government. The War of the Masks in May–June 2020 transformed facial masks from simple devices to block contamination and viral shedding into symbols of political allegiance. Politically put, Democrats were more willing to wear masks in public than Republicans, especially when Trump, against the advice of his own medical experts in the administration, refused to wear a mask.[42] But with a resurgence of COVID-19 cases in states that had previously not had high case numbers, some Republican politicians broke with the president and began to urge their constituents to wear masks.[43] This is interesting, because it suggests that political rhetoric can be changed in response to perceived reality, and something that was made a rhetorical symbol can be returned to its original form and function, to be repurposed, rhetorically, by the same people who originally made it a rhetorical symbol.

However, there may be stages in such rhetorical repurposing. On July 1, 2020, near the same time that some Republican politicians began to approve of masks, Trump was asked about his position on masks during an interview on Fox News Business. He said in part:

> Actually, I had a mask on. I sort of liked the way I looked, OK? I thought it was OK. It was a dark, black mask, and I thought it looked OK. Looked like the Lone Ranger. But, no, I have no problem with that. I think—and if people feel good about it, they should do it.[44]

Thus, before the mask is returned to its original function in a pandemic, there can be a pause, during which the meaning, even the constitutional meaning, of wearing a mask shifts. Here, the perceived negative right to not wear a mask was changed by Trump into the positive right to look like a masked fictional character in movies and comic books that a certain generation remembers from childhood. And if they were drawn to that, well, it was permissible—"if people feel good about it, they should do it."

This amounts to "There's no law against it," a deep principle in American life that one is free to do what the law does not forbid. While many Americans might resist the government ordering them to wear masks in a pandemic, the situation is different if rhetorically framed as a freedom to wear a mask. Of course, this proposal only works so long as there is no law against *not* wearing a mask, and Trump and his followers have been resisting such laws. The sly Lone Ranger rhetorical switch contradicted both what the President of Rhetoric of the United States had earlier suggested by his own refusal to wear a mask and his general opposition to the advice of medical experts for avoiding COVID-19. But it gave the mask-advising Republicans some cover, because if one is free to choose to wear a mask, then one is also free to urge others to choose to wear a mask.

The Lone Ranger rhetoric cannot be said to have been motivated by a desire to promote the common good, because Trump went on with his plan for a celebration on the eve of July 4 at Mount Rushmore, with seven thousand in attendance and without social distancing or mask wearing. But perhaps there is a lesson about positive rights in the Lone Ranger interview. The kinds of institutional changes that would improve the lives of nonwhites and poor whites would be motivated by the compassion of their privileged advocates, as well as recognition and promulgation of their positive rights to such changes. The political opposition to government inauguration of such changes would be very strong, and political rhetoric has spurred a culture-war alignment against them. In his July 4 celebration, Trump labeled the Black Floyd protesters as fascist left-wingers making war on the greatness of the United States by destroying symbols of its history in removing Confederate statues.[45] On the same day, the *New York Times* recognized the George Floyd protests as a movement, perhaps the largest in US history; based on polled data, the number of people who had thus far participated in the protests was between 15 and 26 million.[46]

If a Democratic government were to institute changes involving an emphasis on positive rights for some, such changes would likely be met with the kind of backlash that eviscerated the affirmative action programs that were not even required by the government. However, if there were a way to design such changes not as positive rights for some, but rather as entitlements for all, such changes might have a better chance of acceptance.[47]

4

INEQUALITY AND MARGINALIZATION

"The US has needed a trigger to fully address health care disparities; COVID-19 may be that bellwether event. Why is this uniquely important to me? I am an academic cardiologist; I study health care disparities; and I am a black man."

—Clyde W. Yancy, MD[1]

"We hear politicians say all the time that we have the best health-care system in the world. We have fabulous doctors and health-care facilities, but they're off-limits to a lot of people because of the cost."

—Wendall Potter[2]

"That is disgusting, what is happening on those subway cars . . . It's not even safe for the homeless people to be on trains. . . . No face masks, you have this whole outbreak, we're concerned about homeless people, so we let them stay on the trains without protection in this epidemic of the COVID virus? No. We have to do better than that, and we will."

—Governor Andrew Cuomo[3]

Three kinds of racism have become evident during COVID-19: hearts-and-minds racism; discrimination; institutional racism.[4] Hearts-and-minds racism is the explicit, conscious, and deliberate contempt or hatred for people because of their race. Some think it can be unconscious or indirect, and most believe that hearts-and-minds racism is the "real" meaning of *racism*. Direct racial discrimination of treating some worse because of their race has a long history in the medical system, which may have continued through this pandemic. Institutional racism, or organizational practices continuing from original, legalized hearts-and-minds racism and discrimination (e.g., segregation by law), has made nonwhites more vulnerable to the ravages of COVID-19 than whites. Institutional racism can result in poverty and unequal opportunities for people of color, without explicit intent or laws requiring it. Some examples include the following: if people of color do not have the money for medical insurance, they may have higher rates of untreated illness than whites, because lack of money filters out those who cannot afford medical care; those in poor neighborhoods without access to fresh food may be more prone to preexisting illness; low-paying jobs are often stressful, as well as insecure (and stress predisposes people to illness). These and similar factors have resulted in more existing medical comorbidities in nonwhite compared to white populations during COVID-19.

The idea of institutional racism caught wide public interest after the killing of George Floyd, which was also perceived to be discriminatory in the immediate circumstances—that is, Floyd would not have been treated as he was had he been white. People began to understand that the institution of policing concentrated on African Americans, who were subject to greater surveillance and harassment than whites, because they were already disproportionately imprisoned. But this is a vicious circle, because many are in prison because of higher police attention in the first place and a court system that is biased against nonwhites.

Often, if not usually, victims of racism—that is, members of nonwhite groups—are an integral part of the thriving and bustling economic, political, and social systems of US society. But some nonwhites and other groups are marginalized or not fully integrated into the system. Included on the margins are the elderly, people with disabilities, people incarcerated, and the homeless population. Both those experiencing racism and those marginalized are often poor as well. Overall, the diversity of COVID-19 experience is haunted by income and work inequality. The resilience of some may require the greater vulnerability of others. For instance, when disease cases began to surge in New York City, wealthy residents fled, constituting the unwelcome invasion of the Hamptons, as discussed in chapter 2. A more subtle and pervasive example is the risk taken by delivery persons and store clerks to support the isolation of the privileged.

The United States overall is a rich country, and the temporary stop to "new immigrant labor" imposed by the Trump administration during the pandemic (which followed earlier restrictions on refugees seeking asylum) would normally be part of an arrogant response to extreme economic disparities between those living in the United States and the global poor. But this normal-time inequity is alloyed by the fact that the United States for months has had one-quarter of the world's COVID-19 cases, with one-twenty-fifth its population.[5] The health status of the United States may make it an unattractive destination for many would-be immigrants. But, internally, US economic inequalities have played out in pandemic inequalities. A *Forbes* article on April 1, 2020, was titled "The Rich Are Riding Out the Coronavirus Pandemic Very Differently Than the Rest of Us." Apparently, private jet rentals are in holiday-mode shortage and billionaires have taken to their yachts, luxury bunkers, and out-of-the-way vacation homes.[6] It was reported in March 2020 that wealth and fame bought immediate SARS-CoV-2 testing, while others might wait weeks for results, an inequality that continued throughout the summer of 2020, when delays appeared to be worse than ever.[7] While it is not surprising that rich people would use their resources to take care of themselves, the supply chain and processing of SARS-CoV-2 tests was generally complicated and opaque during the pandemic in 2020.[8]

However, privilege during the COVID-19 pandemic has its own costs for those privileged. Money may buy geographical distance from hot spots and faster medical information in addition to treatment, but money is not a panacea against this paradoxical disaster that drives people apart instead of drawing them together. The privilege of being able to work safely at home is offset for women by quarantine demands that challenge feminist gains. At the same time, both dying alone and giving birth alone are new forms of experience for oppressed and privileged alike.

The foregoing issues and others are more systematically examined as the chapter proceeds through two main sections: inequality and marginalization. The chapter concludes with an overall assessment of how COVID-19 affects everyone, existentially.

INEQUALITY

Racial and Ethnic Inequalities

Before proceeding with a discussion of the impact of COVID-19 on diverse ethnic and racial groups, there is some very good news concerning racial inequality and disease, which ought to be registered. To appreciate that good news, a short account of the history of ideas of race as biological is necessary. Nineteenth-century ideas about human races were racist. Whites were always posited as having superior culture and physical health and beauty. Elite scientists and intellectuals, from the most prestigious academic and social posts, insisted that culture and character were inherited along with biological race. But the twentieth century saw a separation in science between biological race (as hereditary) and culture and history (as experienced after birth).

Another, even more important scientific realization was that there was no basis in biology for the kinds of physical racial distinctions that people make in society. There are greater physical (phenotypical) differences within any particular race than between races. No specific genes for any race were discovered, and older ideas that blood types were associated with race were retired. In addition, it was recognized that criteria for racial identity varied according to time and place, even within the same country and state. The scientists of race had posited between three and sixty distinct races, with no uniform standards of demarcation. The mapping of the human genome may have been the final straw breaking the back of the old biologistic ideas of race. No general genetic basis for different races was found, and a scientific consensus emerged that contemporary humans evolved very quickly from the same small population of about ten thousand in Africa.

If social races are picked out first, biological traits associated with them can easily be found. But that is not the same thing as independent discovery in science of a *taxonomy* of human races. The biological human sciences, which were the same sciences that invented the old idea of race, thereby relinquished it—the concept of race ceased to have scientific validity. Everything about race, including perceived physical distinctions and differences, is a social perception, now recognized by scientists as having social origins. All of this has been called *the social construction of race*.[9]

But even after scientists abandoned the idea of biological race, many in medicine and ordinary life continued to associate social races with illness and disease on a biological basis, because some diseases occurred more frequently in some races. In all cases, it was found that it was not racial identity in itself, but rather accompanying social factors, such as poverty, access to health care, and poor nutrition, that caused disproportionate racial frequencies of illness. During the present pandemic, even though African Americans and Latinx contract COVID-19 more frequently and have higher death rates compared to whites, no one has suggested that this is due to physical factors associated with race in a biological sense. That is, no one has suggested, according to old ideas, that racial differences are biological and inherent—that African Americans and Latinx are biologically predisposed to being harder hit by COVID-19 simply because they are black or Hispanic. Everyone seems to understand that they are made more vulnerable by the social conditions that predispose them to preexisting conditions such as obesity, hypertension, and diabetes. Along with these social conditions are living and working conditions that may maximize chances of contagion due to contact with others. This is a major step forward, and the media and the public deserve a lot a credit for having seamlessly absorbed how racial differences are social constructions!

To continue with this encomium, politically opportunistic slurs against Asians and immigrants from Mexico were not made with implications that Chinese and Mexican individuals are inherently, biologically, predisposed to be SARS-CoV-2 "carriers" but referred to the believed geographical origins of outbreaks. Such references, as slurs, are racist, because of preexisting discriminatory stereotypes associated with people from certain places.[10] And these verbal assaults speak to a deep xenophobia in American culture that continues to thwart international cooperation in a worldwide disaster, but they were not inherently racist. That is, such abuse is not racist in the old, now-false biological sense.

The focus on racism during COVID-19 has been on African Americans, but, as already noted, other nonwhite groups have also suffered disproportionately, and observers are now aware of their circumstances. Latinx Americans have suffered both from the disease and from its economic consequences; Asian Americans have been victimized by overt hearts-and-minds racism; Native Americans have been pressured for taking preventative steps against contagion. We will consider these groups in turn, beginning with African Americans.

African Americans

African Americans have not fared well during COVID-19, and their illness and deaths are the effects of centuries-old inequalities in life that have resulted in the cumulative stress of so-called preexisting comorbidities or diseases that magnify the effects of SARS-CoV-2. Often unrealized is the fact that hypertension, diabetes, asthma, obesity, and heart disease are not simply medical ills but conditions of everyday life and its quality that everyone has come to accept and take for granted as "normal." If the realization of the social construction of race were taken to heart, instead of perhaps superficially accepted as a term of art in academic discourse and then thrown around in politically correct media speak, it might be the first step toward recognizing the injustice of these conditions. The literal fact of a "knee on the neck" that became a metaphor in reactions to George Floyd's death is matched by the literal facts of how the goods of life are not equally available to African Americans in American society. Disparities in income, family wealth, education, life expectancy, and yes, health, as well as safety from law enforcement predators, are not abstract quantities but constant qualities of existence. We all know that these differences are the result of ongoing racism and discrimination. So what is likely to be done about them?

If what is to be done is an urgent question, then continued argument about how much of the past should be made public and taught to schoolchildren may be eclipsed by present inequalities that need to be addressed. Senator Tom Cotton (Republican, Arkansas) proposed in late July 2020 that schools with curricula that centered on slavery as a primary motive for founding the United States and its subsequent success should have decreased federal funding. He also said that slavery was "a necessary evil."[11] There is much to take issue with here, on several intellectual and emotional levels. But the content of education may be a secondary concern given the push and pull about reopening K–12 schools for the fall of 2020. Is it a coincidence that a majority of parents who are people of color (91 percent), especially African Americans, oppose such reopening?[12] Do they know something? According to the *Journal of the American Medical Association* (*JAMA*) on June 29:

> In the US, black people account for 13% of the population, but 24% of COVID-19 deaths where race is known. And blacks, Latinos, American Indians [and Asian Americans] also represent a disproportionate number of cases.[13]

Over two months earlier, *JAMA* had reported the emerging disparities that have not changed. Here is how Clyde W. Yancy, the author of the first epigraph to this chapter, put it:

> In Chicago, more than 50% of COVID-19 cases and nearly 70% of COVID-19 deaths involve black individuals, although blacks make up only 30% of the population. Moreover, these deaths are concentrated mostly in just 5 neighborhoods on the city's South Side. In Louisiana, 70.5% of deaths have occurred among black persons, who represent 32.2% of the state's population. In Michigan, 33% of COVID-19 cases and 40% of deaths have occurred among black individuals, who represent 14% of the population. If New York City has become the epicenter, this disproportionate burden is validated again in underrepresented minorities, especially blacks and now Hispanics, who have accounted for 28% and 34% of deaths, respectively (population representation: 22% and 29%, respectively).
>
> The Johns Hopkins University and American Community Survey indicate that to date, of 131 predominantly black counties in the US, the infection rate is 137.5/100,000 and the death rate is 6.3/100,000. This infection rate is more than 3-fold higher than that in predominantly white counties. Moreover, this death rate for predominantly black counties is 6-fold higher than in predominantly white counties. Even though these data are preliminary and further study is warranted, the pattern is irrefutable: underrepresented minorities are developing COVID-19 infection more frequently and dying disproportionately.[14]

So, this is what the parents know. Not because they have read *JAMA*, but rather because these statistics quantify real, lived experience—what is known directly and indirectly in families and throughout communities. And this is the situation that has so far not been directly addressed during the pandemic. Indeed, the *New York Times* reported on July 29, 2020, that 1.7 million black women were unemployed as a result of COVID-19, with predicted setbacks to family wealth and health, together with toxic stress that is likely to have lasting effects on children.[15]

Latinx Americans

Latinx/Hispanic Americans have not fared as well as other racial or ethnic groups during COVID-19, for several reasons that include extensive work in service jobs as frontline workers, multigenerational households with vulnerable elders, and preexisting poverty. They are also a younger group, with less educational attainment than the total population—about half have a high school degree or less. By April 2020, the Pew Research Center reported that half of Latinx/Hispanics experienced a pay cut or lost a job, in contrast to a third of all American adults. Eight million Latinx were employed in restaurants, hotels, other jobs in the service sector, and food-related processing. The experience of pay cuts and layoffs is not significantly different among foreign and US-born Latinx/Hispanics.[16]

In June 2020, the US Supreme Court ruled that the Trump administration's action to end the DACA (Deferred Action Childhood Arrivals) program was arbitrary and unlawful. Over 800,000 Dreamers reside in the United States, of which 200,000 are essential workers, with 27,000 currently employed in health-care work critical to combating COVID-19. However, this ruling may do no more than buy time. The American Dream and Promise Act that would grant permanent residency to illegal immigrants brought to the United States as children has already passed in the House of Representatives, although its passage in the Senate and signing into law will require a different president.[17] Eighty percent of DACA recipients are from Mexico. President Trump repeatedly attacked immigrants from all origins except Northern Europe, and he was only limited in who gets deported by Court rulings such as this one.

Asian Americans

Physical attacks on Asian-appearing individuals are explicit, violent discrimination. Between March and May 2020, over 1,700 incidents occurring in forty-five states were reported, which included stabbing, beating, shunning, workplace discrimination, and verbal abuse.[18] In addition, there was constant blame and suspicion from Republican rhetoric about the "Chinese" or "Wuhan" virus. "Chinatowns" and other Asian enclaves in urban areas throughout the United States have suffered severe economic loss from the closure of restaurants and other service, leisure, and personal care businesses. The result has been higher unemployment and an uncertain future as the general economy reopens.[19] However, members of some Asian American groups may have knowledge of past epidemics and acceptance of mask wearing, from familial ties to communities in Asian countries.[20]

Native Americans

Native American individuals, tribes, and nations are often overlooked in many scholarly and media discussions of minority groups. Their group status of dependent sovereignty has historically yielded both neglect from the federal government and severe constraints on their political and economic autonomy. This general policy often plays out on local levels as well, where the effects of COVID-19 could be especially horrendous within reservations, given limited medical resources and widespread preexisting comorbidities. Prevention of such disproportionate effects of the disease have been resolutely met by tribal lockdowns, but this has come at the cost of abilities to self-fund vital services. Forty percent of the 574 US tribes have relied on taxes from casinos to finance law enforcement, health care, and education, revenue that has dried up with the closure of casinos. Still, out of the $3 trillion Coronavirus Aid, Relief, and Economic Security (CARES) Act, tribal governments should receive $8 billion for public health.[21]

Some tribes chose prevention beforehand, so that extensive treatment capabilities for an outbreak would not be necessary. In May 2020, the Oglala Lakota people of the Pine Ridge Reservation in South Dakota put up six checkpoints blocking tourists from entering their reservation. The governor gave them forty-eight hours to remove these barriers before sending in the National Guard. The tribe held firm, and the governor did not follow through. In Eagle Butte, on the Cheyenne River Reservation, similar checkpoints were installed. A number of state legislators supported the tribal action. The actions taken by both reservations were preventative given high rates of susceptibility due to preexisting diabetes, obesity, lung disease and heart disease, and low medical care capacity.[22] In May 2020, COVID-19 was not rampant in South Dakota, but with over 8,000 cases and 123 deaths two months later, the actions of the tribes proved prescient.

Women and Children

It is a truism about disasters that women suffer more than anyone, because as caregivers they attend to the welfare of others before their own. For many women who work outside their homes or even pursue careers at home, lockdowns and quarantines have disrupted their work lives. Before COVID-19, feminists widely discussed the "second shift" of housework and child care for women who worked outside the home.[23] During COVID-19, working at home or merely maintaining the home is particularly challenging for mothers of school-age children, because they are also expected to support students in online instruction after schools have closed. Their prospects of regaining the employment they left are not robust. In past disasters, when men who were out of work regained employment, their incomes returned to normal levels much faster than those of women.[24]

There is no evidence that in normal times, the (extreme) medicalization of pregnancy (i.e., that it is a medical and not a natural process) has been effective for maternal and fetal health. The United States has a yearly rate of pregnancy and childbirth mortality of 14 out of 100,000 live births, compared to 9 out of 100,000 in the United Kingdom, where maternity is not medicalized to the same extent.[25] Over decades prior to COVID-19, pregnancy had become progressively de-medicalized for healthy women, with fewer drugs and more social interaction and support during childbirth itself. However, COVID-19 prompted hospitals (along with nursing homes) to bar visitors in order to limit contagion. Such caution for the sake of efficient sanitation is reminiscent of the earlier medicalization of pregnancy and childbirth.

The US medicalization of maternity is one extreme of efficiency concerning motherhood in the United States. At the other extreme is the lack of child care. The lack of a national child-care program creates stress in normal times from the uncertainty many working mothers have about being able to get safe, convenient, and affordable child care. If child care is not available or costs more than income from work, mothers are unable to work. The child-care issue has become more intense due to the tension between reopening schools and fears of COVID-19 risks.

At first, the public was told that children could not catch the virus, but six months into the pandemic, there were increasing reports of child deaths from COVID-19, and toxic-shock vascular-type diseases, with likely cardiac complications. Nonetheless, there emerged an apparent consensus that children under the age of ten did not transmit the virus.[26] In normal times, schools relieve families by providing food and social services as well as child care. During COVID-19, the nationwide lack of convenient, safe, neighborhood child-care facilities—taken for granted as a service for working parents in European cities[27]—becomes magnified as an unnecessary and greatly inefficient deprivation. There is no reason, involving child welfare or parental necessity, for education to be combined with total child care as it now is. Children could be taught in schools and cared for in other facilities that are open at all times. A child-care support program for the children of essential workers in New York City has already been developed, and perhaps this program will provide a model for nationwide facilities.[28]

The cultural reason for the lack of accessible, affordable child care for working mothers is somewhat opaque. Does the evident welcome of women into the workplace entail denial that some are mothers? Is there unresolved ambivalence about the fact that most women with young children need to work to support their families? It does not take a huge leap of imagination to sketch the political sides, or interests, here: Democrats understand that child care remains unobtainable or too expensive for many working women, because there is no state support or economy of scale. Many Republicans and conservatives remain skeptical about the need for women to work and the role of the state in making it easier for mothers to work outside of the home. Such prior politicization of accessible child care has made it easy to politicize school reopenings. It is ironic that the sides have switched. It is now Republicans who want schools reopened so that women can return to work, and Democrats or progressives who are conservative concerning COVID-19 risks! Both sides claim to prioritize child welfare, but it doesn't require the wisdom of King Solomon to decide who is more sincere.

Domestic abuse, or intimate partner violence (IPV), which has mostly female victims, is another effect of COVID-19 on women and children. The United Nations Population Fund estimated that three months of quarantine or sheltering in place would result in a 20 percent rise in IPV. Isolation, stress, financial pressures, joblessness, and higher alcohol consumption predictably correlate with increased and more severe IPV during disasters, and specialists see little reason for this to change during COVID-19. Escape hatches leading to contact with people and organizations outside the home, including friends, family, and shelters, may be closed. Increases in aggression are made more dangerous by increases in gun sales.[29]

MARGINALIZATION

Elderly

Aging in the United States is a process of marginalization, mainly due to retirement from work and slow retreat from life engagement with younger people who are active in society. The effect on those of the sixty million senior Americans who have been taking COVID-19 news seriously has been dreary. Their need for more extreme quarantine, even after reopenings, has increased isolation, as has separation from family members. Grandchildren may stay in touch with Skype or Zoom, but "it's not the same thing." There has been scant unified government effort to reach out to the elderly, although varied local nonprofit organizations have provided food, medical transportation, and bill-paying assistance to many marooned in their homes.[30]

In 2016, 26 percent of Americans over age sixty-five, or twelve million, lived alone.[31] However, as lonely as the effects of COVID-19 are for seniors who have quarantined, the situation has been far worse for those who have contracted it. According to KFF (Kaiser Family Foundation) reporting on July 24, 2020, eight out of ten people who died from COVID-19 were age sixty-five or older. The data include states that have had disproportionate deaths in long-term care facilities where contagion can be rampant.[32] The 80 percent death percentage holds for most data on death from disease—old people are most likely to die. In the case of COVID-19, it is believed that older patients have higher mortality due to preexisting conditions and weaker immune systems in general. Of course, this does not mean that younger people are not at risk. The CDC released this assessment in May 2020:

> We estimated that 45.4% of U.S. adults are at increased risk for complications from coronavirus disease because of cardiovascular disease, diabetes, respiratory disease, hypertension, or cancer. . . . Those at elevated risk include 19.3% of people age 18 to 29 and 80.7% for people over age 80.[33]

President Trump may have blown seniors a dog whistle in light of poll reports of wavering or vanishing support from senior citizens who had voted for him in 2016. Trump, himself age seventy-four, puzzled media pundits by boasting of his ability to remember five words from a standard dementia test he took in 2020—person, man, woman, camera, TV. The ostensible motivation for patting himself on the back in this way was his unfounded claim that Joe Biden, age seventy-seven, at the time ahead of him in polls for the 2020 election, could not do so.[34] But it may also have been a message directed to his erstwhile senior supporters: If they could remember those words, especially in order, as he did, then they shared Trump's amazing mental agility and were brilliant for their age. So—hint, hint, hint, hint, hint—maybe they should vote for him again after all.

Still, even with a Democratic administration, there is dim light at the end of the tunnel for elderly Americans, before the pandemic itself passes or there is herd immunity from an effective vaccine. However, natural or organic herd immunity, in an October 2020 plan attributed to the Trump administration, is a dangerous proposition. Scientists have projected different levels of infection, from 20 to 80 percent, in order to achieve herd immunity, and 60 to 250 million Americans infected would result in about 600,000 to 2.5 million deaths at a current death rate of 1 percent. Moreover, this death rate could be a yearly rate if immunity is not long lasting.[35]

Disabled

People with disabilities had not been fully integrated into US society before COVID-19. They were marginalized by residence in group homes, employment discrimination, lack of accessibility to many amenities, such as public transportation, and general public aversion to their physical persons. According to the Centers for Disease Control (CDC), disability in itself does not make it more likely for people to contract SARS-CoV-2. However, the CDC goes on to note that "those with chronic lung disease, a serious heart condition, or a weakened immune system" are more likely to become infected or have severe COVID-19 illnesses. And "adults with disabilities are three times more likely than adults without disabilities to have heart disease, stroke, diabetes, or cancer than adults without disabilities." In addition, limited mobility or inability to practice social distancing are specific vulnerabilities for those with disabilities, as is difficulty understanding information or being able to communicate their symptoms of illness.[36]

About 61 million Americans, or 26 percent of the population, have a disability of some kind, and 7.37 million, or over 2 percent of the population, have an intellectual or developmental disability. Two aspects of these vulnerabilities, the first individual and the second external, should be noted. Individuals with intellectual disabilities may be unable to understand the basics of COVID-19, such as what a virus is. And those requiring personal care, especially in group home facilities, may experience disruptions in their care, without understanding why the care they are accustomed to is not forthcoming. Externally, the health-care system may be discriminatory against persons with disabilities during the pandemic. In some states, according to modified principles of triage, those with "severe or profound mental retardation" may have restricted access to ventilators, for non-COVID-19-related disorders as well as COVID-19. It has been argued that such restrictions on care violate the Americans with Disabilities Act, because it is based solely on the disability and not the predicted response to treatment.[37] It is important to clarify what this means.

Normal *triage*—for instance, at the scene of an accident—entails that those with serious injuries, from which they could recover if treated, are treated first. Those with minor injuries or fatal injuries are treated later, or not at all. Triage in a pandemic may involve not treating people who are less likely to benefit from treatment when medical supplies are scarce. Starr County Memorial Hospital, in a Texas county on the border with Mexico, with mostly poor Hispanic residents, announced that as result of a surge in cases in July, a "death panel" would be formed to send patients assessed unlikely to benefit from treatment home to die.[38] As brutal as this plan was, it was based on triage within the context of COVID-19 conditions. The prior decision to withhold ventilators from intellectually disabled patients was not based on the medical context of COVID-19, but rather on the fact that they were cognitively disabled—therein lies the discrimination.

Incarcerated

Prisoners are marginalized—literally. The main purpose of the prison system, in addition to punishment, is the removal of convicted criminals from society. Incarceration is a type of exile that occurs within society. Money is made from prison construction and employment. Prisons entail close confinement, limited access to PPE, and higher preexisting respiratory and cardiac comorbidities among inmates. All of these factors are believed to contribute to higher rates of COVID-19 contagion and death in US prisons when compared to the free population.

Data on testing within prisons has not been regularly reported to a central source, although the UCLA Law COVID-19 Project collected daily counts from March 31 to June 6, 2020. By June 6, 2020, there were 42,107 cases of COVID-19 and 510 deaths among 1,295,285 prisoners. This was a case rate of 3,251 per 100,000 prisoners, or 5.5 times higher than the US rate of 587 per 100,000. The death rate was 39 per 100,000 compared to 29 per 100,000. Prisons hold fewer individuals over age sixty-five, and after adjustments for age, as well as sex, the death rate was three times higher than that in the general US population. Data on testing rates was incomplete, although mass testing showed that infection rates were over 65 percent in some facilities.[39] In addition to contagion within stable prison populations, cases may increase due to inmate transfers, as occurred in San Quentin Prison in the summer of 2020. Lack of testing for new admittees, added to lack of quarantine facilities, suggests a grim future.[40] There is no evident discrimination here, except for the way prisoners are housed and an apparent lack of commitment toward making substantial efforts to decrease their vulnerabilities. However, as pertains to disabled Americans, the impact of COVID-19 on those incarcerated may only be accurately reported after the pandemic is past.

Homeless

In the third epigraph to this chapter, the headline about Governor Cuomo's daily briefing on April 3, 2020, suggested disgust at the sight of homeless people sleeping in New York City subway cars, and also as his commitment to do something about it.[41] It was ambiguous whether the governor was disgusted by the sight of the homeless sleeping in subway cars or the fact that they had nowhere else to sleep. The reaction of disgust is common among many middle-class Americans when they encounter homeless people or see them performing biological functions in public. It is easy for those who are housed to be oblivious to the fact that the homeless have no private place in which to sleep, wash, go to the bathroom, and so forth.

The governor first had the subways cleared every night so that they could be disinfected.[42] This raises the question of where the homeless went when they were removed. The City of New York instituted a program with 139 hotels (one-quarter of the hotels in the city) to provide housing for homeless people who could not socially distance in shelters. Reports of the program make it clear that although the program provides much-needed income for hotels that have been devastated by quarantines, lockdowns, and drastically reduced travel, it is a temporary measure.[43] And there is no evidence that it solves housing or social distancing problems for homeless people who are not in shelters.

It is obvious that those who are homeless cannot practice social distancing or quarantine or lockdown, and that they are unable to frequently wash their hands. The US CDC estimates that 1.4 million homeless people a year are housed in shelters (not all the same people, and not at the same time). On May 1, 2020, the CDC reported on the plight of the homeless during the pandemic:

> Overall, 1,192 residents and 313 staff members were tested in 19 homeless shelters. When testing followed identification of a cluster, high proportions of residents and staff members had positive test results for SARS-CoV-2 in Seattle (17% of residents; 17% of staff members), Boston (36%; 30%), and San Francisco (66%; 16%). Testing in Seattle shelters where only one previous case had been identified in each shelter found a low prevalence of infection (5% of residents; 1% of staff members). Among shelters in Atlanta where no cases had been reported, a low prevalence of infection was also iden-

tified (4% of residents; 2% of staff members). Community incidence in the four cities (the average number of reported cases in the county per 100,000 persons per day during the testing period) varied, with the highest (14.4) in Boston and the lowest (5.7) in San Francisco.[44]

The relatively low figures do not count illness or death among homeless people who do not reside in shelters.

Médecins Sans Frontières (MSF), or Doctors Without Borders, is a medical service organization well known for its international work in war zones and other disaster areas outside of the United States. MSF has been working to provide public service information and support local health organizations throughout the world during the COVID-19 outbreak. In the United States, they have provided aid for homeless people in New York City and for migrant workers in Florida.[45] In New York City, MSF provided showers, hygiene products, cell phones, and also portable washing stations.[46] It is perhaps amazing that the United States appears to be the only rich and highly developed nation requiring MSF's services, but it also speaks volumes about national and local incapacities in dealing with the current crisis. Before COVID-19, there had been no effective national or widespread local way to address to the societal condition of homelessness. It remains to be seen whether this situation will change once the more urgent mainstream problems with the pandemic subside.[47] However, the vulnerabilities of the chronic homeless, which are compounded by the pandemic, are not the only problem insofar as further disaster has worsened their plight. In early September 2020, 150,000 homeless people in California were at risk from air pollution caused by wildfires, from which refuge in shelters already posed problems for COVID-19 social distancing.[48]

EXISTENTIAL EFFECTS

It is the universality of COVID-19, how it affects everyone, that constitutes its existential nature. COVID-19 defies the usual expectations and definitions of disaster, whereby people are naturally drawn to go to some "ground zero" as volunteers. Places experiencing surges do receive help from medical personnel who are willing and able to travel. But outside of hospitals and on a quotidian level, COVID-19 has kept people apart. Six-feet social distancing, facial concealment by masks, quarantines and lockdowns, avoidance of large gatherings, and avoidance of any gatherings involving those who are vulnerable, are all engines of isolation. Paradoxically, such isolation is disproportionately "enjoyed" by those privileged enough to work at home or have enough space to practice social distancing or get along without working. Twenty-eight percent of Americans now live alone, but chosen solitude or solitude that develops with changes in normal life circumstances (e.g., divorce, widowhood, the empty nests of single parents) is not the same thing as imposed solitude that is understood to be necessary to reduce risks of serious illness and death.

Many are terrified by the thought of dying alone, whether because of the virus or other illnesses, without family and friends present. Doctors and nurses may fill in, so that the patient is not literally alone, and many have laudably facilitated last FaceTime conversations. But the inability to exchange comforting words and touch, to enact ending reconciliation and say final good-byes in person, constitutes a psychic void. In normal times, according to anecdotal evidence from hospice workers, dying patients surrounded by loved ones often decide to expire when others have left the room.[49] Still, like forced instead of chosen isolation, there is an absence of liberty for terminal COVID-19 patients. Moreover, unlike death in normal times, those who die during the pandemic do not have the reassurance of leaving a world in more or less good shape. They do not know what will happen to their friends, coworkers, and family members, or, for that matter, to the rest of human society. The result is that death may be not only lonely but also fraught with anxiety, so that the "good death," or death with a mind at peace, seems unlikely. For surviving friends and relatives, isolated death during COVID-19 is compounded by attenuated funereal rituals, from memorial services to burials.

Altogether, the separations making up the psychic toll of COVID-19 are *existential*. Everyone experiences them in one way or another and they cannot be escaped until the pandemic is over. Some inevitably lasting changes, such as more reflection and higher valuation placed on human relationships and contact, may be silver linings. But we do not know how many people will be permanently damaged by their experiences of isolation, or whether the habits of isolation, like other trauma-induced habits, will be lasting scars, or how many of those who bounce back will experience post-traumatic stress disorder (PTSD).[50]

All of these problems have lessons about the pre-COVID-19 structure of society that inspire reassessment and could lead to lasting change. The George Floyd/Black Lives Matter protests have created a palpable widespread public demand for police reform. The racism that police reform would address is a combination of hearts-and-minds racism in the attitudes of police officers toward racial minorities, discrimination in how police officers treat nonwhites differently from whites, and institutional racism through the ongoing conditions that make nonwhites more vulnerable than whites to police misconduct. Chapter 5 is a consideration of police reform.

Alterations in the configuration of work and the prestige of now-exploited essential workers may result in higher wages and more respect for the jobs done by those recognized as essential. The institutional racisms and their history, which disadvantage nonwhites, will require carry-through from the twenty-six-million-strong protests in reaction to George Floyd's killing. As yet, there are no movements or new policies to address the ethnic and racial disparities in COVID-19 illness and death, except for individual and community self-help. The deep-rooted feminist issues related to child care could be addressed either by universal, federal, or locally funded nonprofit child care or by a new industry. In either case, there would be local resources for looking after children in smaller groups than those attending schools.

The marginalization of the elderly, those with disabilities, homeless people, and the prison population could be addressed by separating work from identities and making more kinds of jobs available to whoever can do them. Some of these solutions will require government funding, which may not be permanently forthcoming if looming macroeconomic problems are addressed in the present context of capitalist neoliberalism. Or such money may be forthcoming if policy makers and legislators in the United States have a mandate for larger and more finely meshed safety nets, to be financed by a redistribution of income that narrows the gap between rich and poor. Economic problems will be the subject of chapter 7. However, the questions raised by personal alienation and dying are, as noted, deeply existential, and they will linger in literary and theoretical projects throughout the humanities—they cannot be fixed by money from the government.

In addition, while the COVID-19 pandemic is ongoing, it introduces a new known factor concerning death. Everyone is vulnerable to the disease and anyone can die from it. Ordinarily, death is possible for anyone at any time, but from a variety of causes. Death from COVID-19 is the same cause, and this overhanging risk, in sparing no one, is the heart of the nature of the pandemic.

5

POLICE REFORM

"Police officers must act quickly to seize wrongdoers and obtain evidence while protecting themselves and bystanders. It is easy to second-guess their search-and-seizure decisions in a secure courtroom."

—William Barr[1]

"Let me be clear: as I have said repeatedly, I do not believe that all police officers are bad, nor do I believe that most are bad. But there must be a transparent, impartial and fair system to judge those that engage in criminal or unethical acts."

—Al Sharpton[2]

It will be instructive to begin this chapter with the following passage from Ta-Nehisi Coates's *Between the World and Me*:

You may have heard the talk of diversity, sensitivity training, and body cameras. These are all fine and applicable, but they understate the task and allow the citizens of this country to pretend that there is real distance between their own attitudes and those of the ones appointed to protect them. The truth is that the police reflect America in all of its will and fear, and whatever we might make of this country's criminal justice policy, it cannot be said that it was imposed by a repressive minority. The abuses that have followed from these policies—the sprawling carceral state, the random detention of black people, the torture of suspects—are the product of democratic will. And so to challenge the police is to challenge the American people who send them into the ghettos armed with the same self-generated fears that compelled the people who think they are white to flee the cities and into the Dream. The problem with the police is not that they are fascist pigs but that our country is ruled by majoritarian pigs.[3]

Ta-Nehisi Coates is insightful in relating police misconduct to a broader will in society, and the "majoritarian pigs" he refers to would include both the white leaders of society and the members of the public who comply with their orders, demands, and wishes. Of course, not all of these white people specifically will police abuses; rather, they lack the will to stop them. This is a difficult claim because the area of responsibility for the consequences of not doing something is morally gray, especially when it may not be known what one is morally required to do. If viable proposals for police reform are explicitly put before the white public, which they have not generally been, then one could hold those who reject them morally responsible for continued abuses, but in the absence of that, most majoritarians would be blindsided by a charge of responsibility.

With the death of George Floyd, the public was graphically shown injustice with no immediate remedy that they could take. So between fifteen and twenty-six million of them simply took to the streets. And it was natural for them to turn to, and on, those concrete individuals they regularly see who have the dual power of protection and predation. This is why the police became such an important subject in that moment—the police protect by keeping the peace and the police arbitrarily harm. People could see that instead of protection, here was arbitrary harm—even murder. Those who made up the large crowds in public were not suddenly reflecting on their own part in a racist system—as Coates's claim would seem to require—but in many cases coming to their first full realization of the existence of that system. The scales of color blindness slid away.

The George Floyd crowds were racially inclusive and diverse in age, ethnicity, and gender. This suggests that in addition to compassion for the fate of George Floyd and others racially like him, many in these crowds were also themselves victims of systemic oppression, in the present and the past, from the police and from other authorities and institutions in society. That is, unarmed black men who have been executed by police officers are not the only victims of oppression in US society. Here are just a few further examples: Native Americans who suffered removal from their lands and genocide by the US military; women who until recently did not have the right to vote and to this day suffer unchecked violence and sexual harassment; people with disabilities who endure both their disabilities and contempt and neglect from others because of them; immigrants and refugees at all times, including recent cases of children kept in cages at the US southern border; LGBTQ people who experience police brutality in addition to other ambient abuse; white poor people in a prison system that is disproportionately nonwhite, but in which their absolute numbers are highest; homeless people whose most quotidian biological actions are considered crimes because they do not have the privacy of shelter. It should be noted that lists of these groups of oppressed and victimized people include higher numbers of poor whites than poor nonwhites, but that is because whites are overall greater in number than nonwhites. This fact can be taken out of context to minimize harm to nonwhites,[4] which overrides considerations of justice. Injustice is the issue when members of some groups are disproportionately subject to it (for instance, the injustice of a prison system that is almost half black when blacks make up just 14 percent of the overall population).

President-elect Joe Biden has said that the institution of slavery is America's "original sin."[5] This is a narrow view, although it may be necessary rhetoric for a time when race relations come to a crisis. A broader view is that the original sin of the United States, against the context of its stated ideals, is injustice. Not all now and in the past suffer from injustice in the United States. But those who do not suffer from it, and for that reason tolerate others suffering from it, belong in a category similar to what Coates calls "majoritarian pigs," although they may not even be a numerical majority when all of the victims of injustice are added up. If all of those victims were to collectively demand justice, the fifteen to twenty-six million whom the *New York Times* counted as participants in the George Floyd/Black Lives Matter protests would be the avant-garde of revolution—revolution against those in power and those who obey them and tolerate their injustice to others.

This is not the context to interrogate the nature of a people who do not themselves experience injustice and thereby tolerate others' experience of injustice. That context would be the wider context of the historical nature of "we the people" and their culture. Here, the subject is the smaller—but no less perplexing—one of police reform. The first part of

this chapter is about the local structure and culture of US police departments. Next is an examination of the ultimate legal structure protecting
police violence. The chapter ends with possible local solutions, through
community policing.

THE NATURE OF US POLICE DEPARTMENTS

In early July 2020, the Donald Trump campaign released a television
commercial about contacting the police after "defunding." The call was
answered as follows:

> You have reached the 911 police emergency line. Due to defunding
> of the police department, we're sorry, but no one is here to take your
> call. If you're calling to report a rape, please press 1. To report a
> murder, press 2. To report a home invasion, press 3. For all other
> crimes, leave your name and number and someone will get back to
> you. Our estimated wait time is currently five days. Good-bye.

The ad ended with the text, "You won't be safe in Joe Biden's America."[6]

It is fitting that President Trump presented himself as "the law and
order president," and then candidate, in the 2020 election, because the
focus on police misconduct in the midst of COVID-19 USA is a *trope*—
that is, a part representing the whole. Police misconduct, which in the
case of George Floyd's death galvanized millions, can be understood to
exceed its literal self to represent the failure of government to protect
the people. Hence, Trump's rhetorical implication in this message,
complete with "Keep America Great" at the end, is that only he as
president could protect America—but from what, exactly? If the protesters represented enough Americans (which they did if the members
of all groups they represent are counted), then Trump was campaigning
on a platform to protect Americans from themselves. But here is a case
in which rhetorical illogic doesn't really matter, because neither Donald
Trump nor Joe Biden would have the power as president to "Keep
America Safe" in terms of whether police are reformed (or "defunded"). This is because US police departments are neither funded
directly by the federal government or the states nor directly controlled
by these government entities. US police departments are local organiza-

tions. It's important to understand this structure and its cultural implications.

The United States criminal justice system consists of law enforcement, courts, and carceral institutions. Individuals who have been convicted of crimes move through this system, in order, but not all who encounter law enforcement are convicted or incarcerated. Law enforcement or police organizations in the United States consist of federal, state, and local entities with both distinct and overlapping jurisdictions and powers. There are about 18,000 police agencies or departments, including city police departments, county sheriff's offices, state police or highway patrol, and federal law enforcement agencies. All of the law enforcement agencies investigate crime and refer those arrested to municipal, county, state, or federal prosecutors.

Police have duties to prevent and interrupt crimes and serve warrants and other court orders. Police also have obligations of emergency first response and the protection of public facilities and officials, as well as jail detention. Federal police units enforce federal laws and report to government agencies such as the Federal Bureau of Investigation (FBI), Drug Enforcement Administration (DEA), Bureau of Alcohol, Tobacco, Firearms, and Explosives (ATF), the US Marshals Service, the Federal Bureau of Prisons (BOP), and the Department of Homeland Security (DHS). Several agencies also report to DHS: US Customs and Border Protection (CBP), US Immigration and Customs Enforcement (ICE), the Transportation Security Administration (TSA), United States Secret Service (USSS), and the United States Coast Guard (USCG), the latter reporting to the US Department of Defense in war. The United States Park Police (USPP) are part of the National Park Service, which is part of the Department of the Interior (DOI).

Although there are federal police, as part of different federal agencies, departments, and units, according to the US Constitution, the federal government has no national police powers. Each state has a general law enforcement agency and bureau of investigation or department of justice. County, city, and town police agencies may overlap geographically in duties and jurisdiction. The largest may be the New York City Police Department (NYPD), with about 40,000 members; most departments are far smaller. The total number of law enforcement officers in the United States is now 800,000.[7]

A 2019 Pew Research Center survey reported that the majority of black (87 percent) and white (63 percent) Americans believed that police treated blacks less fairly than whites. These percentages are unlikely to have decreased in light of the George Floyd/Black Lives Matter protests.[8] Nevertheless, the organization of police departments, or their culture, tends to be resistant to change. Superintendents or chiefs of police departments are more likely to attribute episodes of violence to rogue officers, rather than to the system or departments that enable them. Proposed reforms that have been published and circulated for more than one hundred years include Community Oriented Policing (COP); the learning and practice of de-escalation skills; greater racial diversity among police officers; better data collection and transparency; and more thorough screening of recruits and hirings across police departments.[9] The last is important because there is a widespread practice of officers with misconduct records in one department being able to simply start fresh in another one. Moving to another state is one way this can be done, and the new department, especially if it is local, may not have the resources to do a thorough background check. Police unions also protect these so-called Gypsy Cops (a slur on Roma people).[10]

Democrats and other progressives are generally pro-labor and thereby pro-union, while Republicans and conservatives are loath to criticize or attack police unions, either because of a general aversion to what would ultimately be legislation representing government interference or for political "law and order" identities and support. However, there is a general consensus that in the absence of other changes, police unions create the strongest barriers to change. Police unions protect members accused of misconduct and have been able to settle internal disputes through arbitration behind closed doors. They are well funded and contribute to political campaigns, which gives them additional clout to pressure lawmakers to block initiatives for investigating or punishing police misconduct. They can sign federal consent decrees but see that their members fail to implement them.

Police unions generally support officers charged with crimes, even in the case of George Floyd's killing. Police union leaders have called protesters "terrorists," and part of the reason for the increase in violent crime following George Floyd's death has been attributed to a nationwide slowdown in police response to law-and-order issues. When Steve Fletcher, a Minneapolis city councilman, tried to divert money from new officer hires to an office of violence prevention, he said of the union regarding slowness in police response to 911 calls, "It operates a little bit like a protection racket."[11]

Legal Support of Police Impunity[12]

The injustice of the murder of black men by police and its relation to racism is very blatant. There is an asymmetry between what counts for just and unjust treatment for groups. For a group to be treated justly, most members or a high proportion of a group need to be treated justly. But for a group to be treated unjustly, it is sufficient if a smaller number, or a lower proportion than required to meet the standard of just treatment, be treated unjustly. The reason for this asymmetry may be that just treatment is easily normalized within communities, whereas unjust treatment of only a few is disruptive and considered abnormal among other members of their group. There is not only the disruption to daily life caused by the unjust treatment of a small number but also a disruption that ripples out from their friends and relations. More problematic, if the group treated unjustly is believed to be treated unjustly because they are not white in white-dominant society, then strong feelings about racism strengthen the indignation.

A basic principle of fairness is continually violated. Immediate moral and emotional reactions that it is *wrong* for police to stop young black men and subject them to humiliating searches without probable cause (that is, they are not otherwise evidently committing crimes) are based on the fact that young white men are not treated that way. When white police officers are not punished for killing unarmed young black men after they have racially profiled them in such ways, it is perceived to be *unjust* according to standards for retributive justice that are routinely upheld when unarmed whites are not arbitrarily stopped and killed. American whites who are innocent of crimes have less to fear from their local police in this regard. There are no high-profile cases of unarmed white teenagers being gunned down for no reason days before they are scheduled to attend college. Should that happen, it would be a terrible mistake, a punishable offense, a disruption that would cause immediate changes in whatever the police policies were, as well as profound apologies to surviving family members from all officials concerned. Along these lines, Michelle Alexander in *The New Jim Crow* writes:

> Can we envision a system that would enforce drug laws almost exclu-
> sively among young White men and largely ignore drug crime among
> Black men? Can we imagine young White men being rounded up for
> minor drug offenses, placed under the control of the criminal justice
> system, and then subjected to a lifetime of discrimination, scorn, and
> exclusion? Can we imagine this happening while [imagining] most
> Black men landed decent jobs or trotted off to college?[13]

Some police officers throughout the United States are racist and abuse their power; other police officers tolerate their behavior; and the public has a long history of tolerating the whole configuration. Video recordings of egregious killings have shocked Americans in recent years but have not stopped racist hate groups from forming and growing, much less ended such killings. I cannot do justice here to the individual killings or the antiracist arguments and pleas that such killings have evoked. George Floyd's death was perhaps the most watched video of death that had ever been viewed, and yet, on the day Floyd died and the days and weeks after, additional incidents of the same nature occurred and were reported in the popular media.[14] Why does this happen? Some police officers are untrained and some are deliberately, consciously racist. It is also likely that some are avowed White Supremacist extremists who have a goal of killing black men. Many members of the public are outraged but have so far been helpless to stop such crimes from recurring.

Forensic expert Lawrence Kobilinsky precisely makes the legal distinction necessary for understanding the requirements for the prosecution of police murder as a crime, noting, "If somebody shoots somebody else, the medical examiner's going to call it a homicide. Now whether it's criminal, is a different story."[15] What I and others have been calling "murder" is in law "criminal homicide," and that charge (accusation) of a death caused by a police officer must be put by a prosecutor before a grand jury before a trial is possible. A very simple pragmatic reason for the recurrence of police killings is that formal charges of murder require extraordinary outrage to be brought, and it is still more rare for convictions and criminal punishment to follow from a trial by jury. Part of the obstacle to indictments is that local police and prosecutors work closely together in the vast majority of other criminal cases that are prosecuted, making it difficult for prosecutors to break these ties in cases involving the prosecution of police officers.[16] Thus, besides not being morally or professionally accountable, police officers are often not found legally accountable (which is to say, indicted and tried for murder).

Worse yet, if every police officer who murdered a suspect was indicted and tried for murder, the widespread practice of not-guilty jury verdicts would likely continue. This is because judges instruct juries on the law relating to findings of guilt for such crimes, and judges are bound by higher-court—especially the US Supreme Court—rulings on what the law is. While constitutional and statute law is explicit about equal rights, police discretion and immunity have been protected by US Supreme Court judges. Three important US Supreme Court cases have set precedent: the 1968 opinion in *Terry v. Ohio*; the 1989 opinion in *Graham v. Connor*;[17] and the 2013 ruling in *Plumhoff et al. v. Rickard*.[18] Many high-profile police killings have been the result of "stop and frisk" practices gone bad. Each year, US police departments voluntarily report "justifiable police homicides" to the FBI, which is considered an incomplete record. Out of 2,600 justifiable homicides reported from 2005 through 2011, forty-one officers were charged with murder or manslaughter.[19] Federal agencies have not updated this data since 2014. The *Washington Post* has reported over five thousand police killings between 2015 and 2020.[20] The reason the number of these indictments is low and may continue to be low may rest on these US Supreme Court rulings that have become settled law.

The decision in *Graham v. Connor* is important, because it specifies something other than constitutional rights as a standard for what police officers may not do to individuals. Graham, a diabetic, asked his friend Berry to drive him to a convenience store to purchase orange juice. Graham saw that the store was crowded and hurried out again. Officer O'Connor thought that Graham's movements were suspicious and asked him and Berry to wait while he checked the store. Backup officers arrived and handcuffed Graham, causing injuries. Graham sued, claiming that excessive force had been used in violation of his Fourteenth Amendment rights (to equal protection under the law).

The Court held that all claims that enforcement officials have used excessive force must be analyzed under the "objective reasonableness" standard of the Fourth Amendment (freedom from unreasonable search and seizure), rather than a substantive due process standard requiring that "all government intrusions into fundamental rights and liberties be fair and reasonable and in furtherance of a legitimate government interest." The Court framed the objective reasonableness standard in *Graham* on

> whether the officers' actions are "objectively reasonable" in light of the facts and circumstances confronting them, without regard to their underlying intent or motivation. The "reasonableness" of a particular use of force must be judged from the perspective of a reasonable officer on the scene, and its calculus must embody an allowance for the fact that police officers are often forced to make split-second decisions about the amount of force necessary in a particular situation.[21]

US police academies systematically teach "Graham Factors" for determining when lethal force may legitimately be used: How severe is the crime? Does the suspect pose an immediate threat to the safety of officers and others? Is the suspect resisting arrest or trying to flee?[22]

This recourse to what in other situations might be called the "subjective judgment" of police officers was strengthened in *Plumhoff et al. v. Rickard*. The US Supreme Court ruled in 2013 that individuals' Fourth Amendment rights violations must be balanced against an official's *qualified immunity*, unless it can be shown that the official violated a statutory or constitutional right that was "clearly established" at the time of the challenged conduct.[23]

Both *Graham* and *Plumhoff* constitute a change from a focus on the constitutional rights of citizens against unreasonable (that is, unprovoked and unwarranted) search and seizure to what it seems "reasonable" for a police officer to do in the heat of the moment. Many Americans still believe that police officers are constrained to behave in ways that make the use of deadly force "a last resort." They may believe that the legal world is still governed by the 1984 US Supreme Court ruling in *Tennessee v. Garner*, where the Court wrote, "The use of deadly force to prevent the escape of all felony suspects, whatever the circumstances, is constitutionally unreasonable."[24] By contrast, at this time, given *Graham* and *Plumhoff*, if "suspicious" people try to flee, it can be construed as "reasonable" that police officers kill them, because once labeled "suspicious," a police officer can reason that the suspect poses a danger to other members of the community. Moreover, if police officers fear for their lives, then it becomes legally reasonable that they resort to deadly force, because, according to the Court, their "underly-ing intent and motivation" are irrelevant to that standard.

The context of "stop and frisk" itself is the factor enabling the cur-rent uses of deadly force that so many consider unjust. To understand the legality of that context, we need to go back to Chief Justice Earl Warren's 1968 opinion in *Terry v. Ohio*. Warren first distinguished between "stops" and "arrests" and between "frisks" and "searches": "stops" are brief police interrogations based on suspicion, and "arrests" are taking suspects into custody based on criminal evidence; "frisks" are determinations of whether the suspect has a weapon, restricted to superficial searches or "pat downs" of the surface of the body, undertak-en for the officer's immediate safety, whereas "searches" are more inva-sive investigations that can be performed only after arrests. Mindful of the exclusionary rule requiring that criminal evidence be obtained law-fully, before an arrest, the Court narrowed its attention to "whether it is always unreasonable for a policeman to seize a person and subject him to a limited search for weapons unless there is probable cause for an arrest."

Warren went on to find that the Fourth Amendment protection against unreasonable searches and seizures applied as much to stops and frisks as to arrests and searches: "We therefore reject the notions that the Fourth Amendment does not come into play at all as a limita-tion upon police conduct if the officers stop short of something called a 'technical arrest' or a 'full-blown search.'" Warren then answers the question of how a Fourth Amendment intrusion is to be justified, with a "reasonable person" standard:

> The scheme of the Fourth Amendment becomes meaningful only when it is assured that at some point the conduct of those charged with enforcing the laws can be subjected to the more detached, neutral scrutiny of a judge who must evaluate the reasonableness of a particular search or seizure in light of the particular circumstances. And in making that assessment it is imperative that the facts be judged against an objective standard: would the facts available to the officer at the moment of the seizure or the search "warrant a man of reasonable caution in the belief" that the action taken was appro-priate?[25]

Warren recognizes that the government has a general interest in crime detection and concludes, based on that interest, that "a police officer may in appropriate circumstances and in an appropriate manner approach a person for purposes of investigating possibly criminal behavior even though there is no probable cause to make an arrest." Furthermore, "It does not follow that because an officer may lawfully arrest a person only when he is apprised of facts sufficient to warrant a belief that the person has committed or is committing a crime, the officer is equally unjustified, absent that kind of evidence, in making any intrusions short of an arrest."[26]

Given the ultimate strength of legal support from the US Supreme Court, the law remains on vacation concerning racial bias in stops of black suspects, as well as racial bias that may exaggerate the perceived danger posed by black suspects in the minds of police officers during episodes of physical confrontation. If, as Warren stated, the interests of the government in preventing and detecting crime may override Fourth Amendment rights in actions by police in stops and frisks, does the same apply to attempted stops and frisks?

The reasonable officer standard may result in legally justified homicide if a police officer fears for his life, even if the officer has used bad judgment in creating a situation in which he put his life in danger. For example, Officer Christopher Manney shot Dontre Hamilton fourteen times after getting into a violent struggle with him in a downtown Milwaukee park in April 2014. Earlier, employees at a nearby Starbucks had called in a complaint against Hamilton for sleeping on a park bench. Two other police officers had responded before Manney arrived and decided that no further police action was necessary. Manney was fired for incompetence in creating the altercation, but it was announced in December 2014 that no charges would be filed against him, because his actions were appropriate after he had created that altercation—that he created it was apparently irrelevant.[27]

Returning to the opinion in *Graham*, underlying intent and motivation are not irrelevant to how human beings behave when race is involved. Beneath the law, or alongside it, in the category of what the US Supreme Court considers irrelevant to the "reasonable officer" standard, anti-black racism, as visceral or bodily and emotional, continues to operate. Racism as emotional and embodied is not a system of beliefs but a system of reaction that may occur faster than and preempt conscious and law-abiding beliefs.[28]

Whether there will be changes in how police homicide is dealt with by the US Supreme Court remains to be seen. Much precedent would have to be dismantled or overturned, which does not seem likely in an increasingly Conservative and conservative (that is, both politically and jurisprudentially progress-averse) Supreme Court. But there can be change in local police practices, leading to fewer arbitrary police homicides. This will mean that judicial decisions are less important than local practices and procedures as a fulcrum for change. Enough local change can add up to national change.

LOCAL SOLUTIONS

The militaristic structure of police agencies, which generates identities as warriors, together with job requirements of expected numbers of stops and arrests, is an obstacle to change from within.[29] This structure generates a culture of violence toward suspects that does not easily self-correct, and it is protected by unions and the courts. For change to occur in police violence and perceived unfairness to people of color, in the absence of changes in US Supreme Court case law, there would need to be internal organizational and cultural changes within local police departments. Community policing, or Community Oriented Policing (COP), is designed for such change. The basic idea of community policing is that instead of police officers imposing orders from above on the communities in which they work, they recruit assistance and information from members of those communities. The interface between officers and community members should thereby be collaborative and cooperative rather than confrontational. In 2013, the Chief Justice Earl Warren Institute on Law & Social Policy at the UC Berkeley School of Law assessed the previous ten years of community policing and defined it as follows:

> More direct officer involvement with local citizens was organized around less rigid hierarchies and protocols, and attempted to address the root causes of neighborhood crime with the assistance of the larger community. Adoption of the community policing philosophy by local police departments occurred gradually throughout the 1970s

and 1980s, and by the early 1990s, more and more cities were beginning to adopt community policing approaches. After decades of
adoption at the local level, community policing was effectively
endorsed by the federal government with the passage of the Violent
Crime Control and Law Enforcement Act of 1994. This bill authorized an initial six-year expenditure of $8.8 billion in federal aid to
support community policing efforts and created the Office of Community Oriented Policing Services (COPS) to distribute and monitor
this funding. Today, the COPS Office continues to operate community policing initiatives nationwide and distribute grant funds to localities to support those efforts. [30]

Studies of the implementation of community policing suggest that officers involved in such programs are generally enthusiastic about them, a
reaction that holds in small- and medium-sized, as well as large, cities. [31]

Plans for community policing support have been put forth by the
federal government, but implementation remains with the states, and it
is not always exactly known how or if federal funding will be forthcoming. During the Obama administration, in May 2015, ten US cities
reported success after enacting community policing programs in
2012. [32] In early June 2020, the Trump administration recommended
eliminating Community Relations Services and Community Oriented
Policing Services and moving their functions to other parts of the Department of Justice. (The combined cost of these programs was less
than $300 million.) [33] After Democrats objected, less than two weeks
later, the Trump administration issued "An Executive Order on Safe
Policing for Safe Communities" that reiterated the need for police certification and training for dealing with homelessness, mental illness, and
other community problems. During the George Floyd protests, the
Trump executive order delegated implementation to the states, and it is
too soon to tell how or if it will be implemented. [34]

The transition from concentration on the legal structure to local
solutions entails an interesting disciplinary or meta-subject shift from
studies of the law to social science/public policy. Along these lines, it
becomes important to track current events and their results as they are
reported, because this is a pressing issue that may take a while for
experts to comprehensively study and quantify. In this spirit, Camden,
New Jersey, a city that has been heralded for successfully implementing
a community policing policy, is worth considering. In 2013, Camden

(population 74,000) was strapped for cash and had the highest crime rates in the nation. Working with the governor, the mayor fired the entire police force and later rehired half of them at reduced pay. New recruits were told that their jobs would more resemble work in the Peace Corps than Special Forces. Crime and complaints of police violence have since decreased. Problems of communication and fines for small offenses persist, and the white police force does not live in the neighborhoods they patrol. Nevertheless, the following incident was reported in 2015:

> The officers encountered the man on the sidewalk outside. Instead of shooting him or trying to disarm him, they walked with him for several minutes. "Drop the knife. Sir, drop the knife," one of the officers said repeatedly.
>
> They tried to disable him with a stun gun, but that failed. Still, the officers managed to tackle the man to the ground and disarm him, apparently without causing serious injury.
>
> "There is not a shadow of a doubt in my mind that six months prior to that, we would have shot and killed that man," said [Chief of Police] Scott Thomson, who retired last year. "That was a watershed moment for our organization. And that was a moment in time that really signaled to me that the cops got it right."[35]

At the end of the conclusion in my 2015 book, *White Privilege and Black Rights: The Injustice of U.S. Police Racial Profiling and Homicide*, I wrote, "Cultures change in small unnoticed ways over varied periods of time and then they can change overnight."[36] I included "and then they can change overnight" because I wanted to end on a note of hope that was nonetheless guarded. I did not envision that the bleak situation of nationwide, unpunished police crime—which was unpunishable because of the legal foundation the US Supreme Court had provided—was likely to change overnight. So the *can* was a reference to possibility. But it is known from local examples that such changes are possible. There may be a will for them to spread, so that they can become national. In other words, for a number of reasons, COVID-19 may have brought the United States to long-needed police reform.

The obstacles, in the organizational structure of police departments, settled law from the US Supreme Court, the power of police unions, and Republican politics, are depressing. In a 2019 event study (with robust controls) of the number of police killings of civilians following 700 mass protests about police violence against African Americans during the 1960s and early 1970s, Jamein Cunningham and Rob Gillezeau found discouraging results:

> Historical protest resulted in an increase in civilian deaths by legal intervention regardless of race in the short run and a seemingly permanent increase in killings of non-white[s] over the medium to long run. These results paint a depressing picture in which uprisings represent a structural change in police–civilian relations, adversely affecting white civilians in the short run and non-white civilians in the short and long run.[37]

However, the racially inclusive nature of the George Floyd/Black Lives Matter protests this time, as well as their widespread support by business and social organizations, plus the ongoing development of Community Oriented Policing, may be grounds to hope that we are on the brink of all-at-once change. Such hope is supported by the commitment to racial justice by President-elect Biden and Vice President-elect Harris.

6

EDUCATION

"The good Education of Youth has been esteemed by wise Men [*sic*] in all Ages, as the surest Foundation of the Happiness both of private Families and of Commonwealths [nations]. Almost all Governments have therefore made it a principal Object of their Attention, to establish and endow with proper Revenues, such Seminaries of Learning, as might supply the succeeding Age with Men [*sic*] qualified to serve the Publick with Honour to themselves, and to their Country."

—Benjamin Franklin[1]

"Change is the end result of all true learning."

—Leo Buscaglia[2]

"You ask me about the idiosyncrasies of philosophers? There is their lack of historical sense, their hatred of even the idea of becoming . . . nothing actual has escaped from their hands alive. They kill, they stuff, when they worship, these conceptual idolaters—they become a mortal danger to everything when they worship."

—Friedrich Nietzsche[3]

Education in the abstract is knowledge and skills that can be taught and learned. But as part of society, education is a group of institutions, not necessarily united, but serving common purposes. The purposes include social instruction, interaction, and positioning, as well as certification of the acquisition of certain kinds of knowledge and skills. There are two main educational groups in the United States: K–12 and higher education. Apart from grades that usually must be completed to advance to the next grade and prior degrees required to study for more advanced ones, the unity between these groups or among their members is based on general standards to which they individually adhere or subscribe. Public K–12 schools are rooted in distinct geographical neighborhoods, so that their students share residential areas. Institutions of higher education may serve counties, states, or regions, but except for community colleges, they are less tied to where students reside with their families. In most instances, on different levels, schools are not connected to one another except for special scholarly or athletic events. Still, despite these distinctions and institutional autonomies, it makes sense to speak of "the American educational system," which means that there are deep commonalities of function and service. And, in addition to this educational system, which is largely a "retail" apparatus, there is the dimension of research that ultimately determines the content of the whole system. Research in the sciences is funded by the federal government, corporations, and educational institutions, and much of it is physically conducted on college campuses.

In order to understand the impact of COVID-19 on education in the United States, it is necessary to begin with some general, quasi-official facts and numbers to grasp the magnitude of what is at stake. This is the first section of the chapter. Next, the societal function of retail education and the contribution of research are considered. At the end, there are lessons for both surviving the pandemic and perhaps improving the educational system.

FACTS AND NUMBERS

Elementary, middle school, and high school education in the United States cost about $1.3 trillion. Most of this funding comes from state and local governments, and the federal government contributes about $200 billion. Eighty-seven percent of all students attend public schools, 10 percent attend private and foundation-funded schools, and 3 percent are homeschooled. The total enrollment for 2020 is 56.4 million students. State laws make education compulsory between the ages of five and eight to sixteen and eighteen. In 1929–1930, there were 248,000 public schools in the United States, but consolidation decreased that to about 98,000 in 2015–2016 (which includes an increase of about 16,000 schools since 2007). According to the Organisation for Economic Co-operation and Development, the United States has the most expensive educational system in the world, but the overall knowledge and skills of American fifteen-year-olds, in reading, literacy, mathematics, and science, is thirty-first in the world. It is important to note here that money spent on education is not the only factor in being able to impart knowledge and skills, although the present focus is not K–12 reform.

There are a variety of postsecondary schools, including highly selective universities, public universities, private liberal arts colleges, historically black colleges and universities, Hispanic-serving colleges, Native American colleges, community colleges, and for-profit distance-learning colleges. Eight of the top ten colleges and universities in the world are in the United States (the remaining two are Oxford and Cambridge, in the United Kingdom). There are 6,606 institutions of higher education, of which 4,360 grant degrees. Of degree-granting institutions, 2,863 are four-year schools and 1,538 are community colleges. Fall enrollment in degree-granting institutions increased 26 percent between 1997 and 2007 and then decreased by 2017, for a total of more than 18 million. About two-thirds are students in four-year institutions. In 2016–2017, the total expenses of degree-granting institutions were $584 billion: $372 billion at public institutions, $197 billion at private nonprofit institutions, and $15 billion at private for-profit institutions. The total endowment of US colleges and universities is almost $600 billion, not counting the value of their real estate assets, which varies according to the national and local markets.[4]

Academic research supports health-care delivery within academic medical centers. Additional research spending in higher education in the United States represents about $74 billion, or 13 percent of the almost $600 billion spent nationally on research. Research institutions are also among the top five employers in forty-four US states, employing 560,000 people plus over 300,000 trainees through research funds.[5]

To sum up, there is a total of close to seventy-five million students in the United States, and close to $2 trillion is spent on their education. This yearly expenditure compares with the market capitalization of the Apple corporation as the first US company to be valued at $2 trillion, on August 19, 2020 (a figure that is a total value of Apple's stock, and as such, subject to change).[6] Insofar as the expenditures of US colleges and universities are planned yearly and are based on endowment income and tuition, their yearly budgets are subject to both enrollment fluctuations and the changing value of their endowments, which are based on financial markets and the overall economy. That is, although higher degree–granting education is not a for-profit business, its finances are subject to inflows of money from students as consumers, donors as funders, and market forces, which altogether constitute a businesslike dynamic.

The gross national product (GNP) of the United States, prior to COVID-19, was about $20 trillion, and the population was about 330 (328.2) million. We can conclude that education is a substantial part of US productivity—close to 20 percent of the population and 10 percent of the GNP.[7] The US GNP is projected to contract over 2020 as a result of the COVID-19 pandemic, and this issue will be discussed in chapter 7. Here, we should note that going into the pandemic, substantial numbers of people and moneys spent on them were at stake in the overall educational system. And in addition to the economic facts, the huge cultural, social, and sometimes political influence of higher education make it a major institution in contemporary society. But although higher education, especially in its research and student activist dimensions, weighs in as an important societal influence, we should not forget that no one gets admitted or certified without having first gone through K–12.

It is well known that individual life earnings increase with education. And insofar as these earnings contribute to GNP, it seems a safe assumption that a robust educational system contributes substantially to national wealth, as well as to individual well-being—the American dream typically unfolds after college graduation. This happens in two ways: the proportion of any present GNP to which the educational system contributes; and future contributions to the GNP and overall individual well-being that the present educational system makes possible as its graduates move through society. If the educational system contracts during COVID-19, which generally seems to be happening, this situation will constitute unpredictable contractions in future GNP and overall individual well-being, depending on the size of the contraction and how much of the educational system can be recovered or productively revised after the pandemic.

To get a sense of how this might work, it's important to understand the pre-COVID-19 societal functions of education and the ways that education could be improved in terms of lessons learned from the pandemic. But before that, if possible, some sense should be made of the disparate and chaotic process of school reopenings for the 2020–2021 academic year.

From February to March 2020, most of the US educational system (i.e., the largest part that was not already online) was simply shut down. According to *Education Weekly*:

> Eventually, 48 states, four U.S. territories, the District of Columbia, and the Department of Defense Education Activity ordered or recommended school building closures for the rest of their academic year, affecting at least 50.8 million public school students. . . . The magnitude and speed of the closures was unprecedented.[8]

Primary, secondary, and college students could no longer go to their campuses for school. Some staff and faculty were furloughed or fired, and those who could work from home were instructed to do that, without disruption to their incomes. Essential security and maintenance staff continued to report for work, to keep physical plants and equipment going, and for cleaning; on most college campuses, outdoor grounds work and landscaping continued. In-person graduation ceremonies were canceled, and the shutdown continued over the summer of 2020. Morale among teachers plummeted as they scrambled to provide online learning and students missed school even if they were technologically equipped to continue from home.[9] This blow to the US educational system had effects that in themselves qualify for disaster designation.

On July 10, 2020, the American Academy of Pediatrics (AAP) issued a complex news statement that sought to balance safety against the need to reopen schools. First, the AAP related the importance of schools to contemporary issues of social equity:

> We recognize that children learn best when physically present in the classroom. But children get much more than academics at school. They also learn social and emotional skills at school, get healthy meals and exercise, mental health support and other services that cannot be easily replicated online. Schools also play a critical role in addressing racial and social inequity. Our nation's response to COVID-19 has laid bare inequities and consequences for children

that must be addressed. This pandemic is especially hard on families who rely on school lunches, have children with disabilities, or lack access to Internet or health care.

But then the AAP deferred to safety concerns.

> Returning to school is important for the healthy development and well-being of children, but we must pursue re-opening in a way that is safe for all students, teachers and staff. Science should drive decision-making on safely reopening schools. Public health agencies must make recommendations based on evidence, not politics. We should leave it to health experts to tell us when the time is best to open up school buildings and listen to educators and administrators to shape how we do it.

And, finally, the AAP emphasized the need for local autonomy, based on differences in COVID-19 outbreaks.

> Local school leaders, public health experts, educators and parents must be at the center of decisions about how and when to reopen schools, taking into account the spread of COVID-19 in their communities and the capacities of school districts to adapt safety protocols to make in-person learning safe and feasible. For instance, schools in areas with high levels of COVID-19 community spread should not be compelled to reopen against the judgment of local experts. A one-size-fits-all approach is not appropriate for return to school decisions.[10]

This local autonomy has resulted in tension between teachers and parents who emphasize the need for underserved children to attend school and those who are immediately concerned about viral contagion. At the beginning of the fall 2020 semester, this situation was further complicated by what remained unknown about viral contagion and the effects of SARS-CoV-2 on K–12 children.[11]

Overall, it seems clear that the AAP collectively believes COVID-19 will determine how and when schools reopen, although it leaves the assessment of risk from COVID-19 up to local officials and individual parents. This idea that "the virus will determine X" became a refrain from health experts, taken up strongly by Democrats, in the fall of 2020, particularly regarding reopening the economy. One important difference between K–12 and higher education is that decisions about re-opening are more centralized in higher education. Administrators of individual private and state system institutions have the power to determine reopening and reclosing in ways that leave less for parents to decide. In most school districts, K–12 parents have options of not sending their children back to school, against the backdrop of compulsory primary and secondary education.

College attendance is not mandatory, so on the "consumption" side, it can be avoided completely, while on the "production" side there is more control. And there has been more control than in other institutions, according to guidelines from the Centers for Disease Control and Prevention and the American College Health Association.[12] (One strange result has been that those campuses usually attended by underserved students, but closed since March 2020, have become beautiful, exclusive, and privileged uninhabited oases for the few administrators and essential personnel who have ongoing access to them. Access is by appointment only, after appropriate training courses have been taken.)

Scholarly work and research in higher education was disrupted as travel to conferences became sharply curtailed. Access to laboratories was restructured according to pandemic safety concerns. Research in the life sciences followed hospital care to focus primarily on COVID-19 and SARS-CoV-2.[13] Overall, research has been ramped down and mitigation and safety guidelines remain works in progress for limited re-openings.[14]

SOCIETAL FUNCTIONS OF EDUCATION

Schools function socially and materially, and they serve wider hierarchical interests in the outside society while benefiting their students as individuals. For example, even within public schools, social status hierarchies among students reflect the status of their parents in the local community. Private K–12 schools charge tuition that only a minority of families can afford. Prestigious and rich colleges and universities have disproportionate enrollment by students from prestigious and rich families. Public colleges and universities have a broader enrollment because they are cheaper to attend, as well as less prestigious—that is, lower in status. There are many complex studies in support of these claims, but here it is sufficient to rely on what everyone already knows: Prestigious colleges and universities cost more than the families of most public school students, especially racial minorities, can afford (average yearly tuition and fees at the eight Ivies is about $56,000).[15] There are scholarships based on merit and need, and many institutions continue to value diversity now that explicit affirmative action has been dismantled by the US Supreme Court. However, the process of being able to successfully apply to top colleges and universities is in itself an inequality that calls for equity. There are admissions tests on two levels: college admission and good preparatory high school admission.

Recently, a small number of rich celebrities were caught spending hundreds of thousands of dollars on bribes and cheating to secure their children's admission into top schools. These parents were arrested, perp-walked, sentenced to prison, and fined.[16] However, to focus on these miscreants would be to miss how privilege is baked into the college admissions process, in perfectly legal ways. There has been plenty of publicity concerning how college admissions tests are culturally biased in favor of white middle-class students, and many institutions have found ways to take this fact into account in support of diversity on college campuses.[17] But often neglected is the fact that successful scores on these tests require preparation. The expense of relevant prep courses is beyond the family budgets of most poor and minority students.

A local example helps spell out the obstacles in this system: New York City has a small number of specialized high schools whose graduates have strong opportunities to attend prestigious and high-quality colleges and universities. In the 1970s, admission tests for these schools required no particular preparation by middle school students. However, since then, students have been required to take a specialized test for admission to these schools. Black and Hispanic students have not scored as well as white and Asian students, and their enrollment has plummeted: Stuyvesant High School went from 14 percent black and Hispanic enrollment to 4 percent; Brooklyn Technical High School, from 50 percent to 14 percent; and Bronx High School of Science, from 23 percent to 9 percent. Success on the specialized test is competitive, and it has come to depend on professionally assisted preparation that has become its own industry. At Kaplan, a leader among the top prep chains, a basic prep course for the New York City specialized school exam costs $1,000 for eight group prep sessions. Most black and His-panic families cannot afford this course, and if their children would be the "first" to attend college, they may not even understand why it is necessary.[18]

Just these general remarks and the New York City example scratch enough of the surface to show that the American educational system, which is not a coordinated, cohesive system, nevertheless reflects and reinscribes status and power structures outside of its walls. While edu-cation remains a primary means for socioeconomic advancement, most graduates return to the status of their families of origin; compared to other countries, there is relatively little upward socioeconomic mobility in the United States.[19] Insofar as the educational system is widely re-garded as the main mechanism for upward mobility, the restrictions for entry into higher education would stabilize social rigidity. It is therefore not surprising that COVID-19 has had differential effects on US educa-tional institutions, depending on their resources before the pandemic. We know, for example, that school districts that were already under-funded find it more difficult to continue their educational missions during the pandemic than those with prior reserves and abundant re-sources.[20] And this situation has had a direct effect on students, accord-ing to the goods and services they depended on before the pandemic. Many students depended on public schools for food, safety, and medi-cal care before COVID-19, and while schools remain closed, these ben-efits have been subject to stopgap measures.[21]

As schoolchildren have returned to school under restrictions during the fall of 2020, there have been dire warnings about the impossibility for many of them to catch up on lost academic time, as well as experi-ences of social development. Children with disabilities who require intensive interactions have suffered extreme deprivation. Many chil-dren succumb to feelings of loneliness, helplessness, and depression if their households are unable to support online learning (or even if they are). Racial minority and poor children fare the worst.[22] Spring 2020 economic modeling based on statistics from World War II school clo-sures suggests that over time, four months of missed education can add up to $2.5 trillion, or 12.7 percent of the US GNP.[23]

The twelve million who attend four-year institutions are involved in an important cultural process that involves living on or near college campuses, at least during the first two years. Campus residence for college students is only superficially analogous to full-day attendance for K–12 students. Being away from home at college fulfills or promises to fulfill the idea of a way of life that will be foundational for the rest of life. They attend for a number of reasons, which they may not be willing or able to clearly articulate: because it is expected of them by family and friends; a desire to leave home as a geographical place; a desire get away from parental supervision and surveillance; a desire to meet new people; a desire to party and/or consume alcohol and drugs; a desire to become part of a fraternity or sorority; a desire to develop and explore their sexuality; attainment of a college degree as a mark of status; attainment of a degree from a particular college; a goal of developing intellectually or acquiring specific knowledge and skills; a goal of participating in a college sport; a goal of a well-paying or fulfilling job that their college degree will make possible; a goal of further education beyond the four-year course of study. These reasons divide into anticipation of the college experience itself and future advantages of having completed that experience. The traditional four-year undergraduate college experience ends with graduation and cannot be duplicated, because its social aspects are age-specific for a time of life without adult responsibilities or settled attitudes toward life.

Not only do college students acquire the knowledge and skills that are formally taught, but they also have opportunities to refine or change their tastes as consumers and learn new habits for lifestyle and recreation. They build up their cultural capital, as well as their social capital from people they meet, befriend, and form networks with.[24] There are clear benefits from having a college degree, in terms of the formal certification and knowledge and skills acquired in college that are qualifications for employment and further study. Such benefits can be quantified by social scientists. But there are other benefits or effects in terms of social position or what used to be simply understood as social class, which are part of the undergraduate experience in ways that require physical presence on campus.

Four-year colleges are partly in the hospitality and recreation business. It is this aspect of what they provide that has made the issue of when and how schools will reopen so fraught. For intelligent young people who have already jumped through the hoops necessary for admission, knowledge and skill learning could take place online, and that would be the end of the story. We would take it as a lesson from

COVID-19 that a college education can be streamlined to what can be delivered and experienced virtually, streamlined to the kernel of its content. But many would find this stark and bleak, a kind of stripping away of the quality of college life which is not mere adolescent sociality but projects of learning about one's peers and inchoately planning the future with them—college friends can go on to do great things together or be inspired later on when they hear about one another's accomplishments in the world after college.

Most of this process is ineffable. But, to put it crudely, college life on or near campus sets up the future class system, occupation of the hierarchies of power to come, and the shared values that will both unite and divide the nation. To consider how this process works, we need consider only two aspects of class in contemporary society: consumption and politics. Consumption becomes a matter of taste during the years of college, consisting of choices in food, clothing, and leisure activities that distinguish those who made them while they were at college from the tastes of those who did not attend college. There are also tastes in music that can ground nostalgia for a lifetime. Political views that arise out of cultural experiences, such as ideas about gender, the importance of addressing climate change, protection of immigrants, and racial justice become generally formed. Insofar as these kinds of political views arise out of common cultural experiences, they were on display during the COVID-19 George Floyd/Black Lives Matter protests.

The cultural and political perspectives that can coalesce while young people are at college show how politics can grow out of the sociality of college culture in ways that bypass both family views and traditional politics, such as the ideological hoopla of elections. These perspectives are the foundation of the so-called culture wars, but, more than that, they have the ability to ground ideas of life for the middle classes of successive generations. However, for college students, a generation is no longer a familial grandparent-child-grandchild progression, but rather a continuously rolling process from entry to graduation, over a course of four years, that leaves the cohort fully occupied with new members. College curricula build on standards for high school curricula, and, to some extent, except when new subjects (e.g., philosophy and anthropology) are introduced, there is cognitive continuity. But the transmission of college culture is not a continuation of high school culture.

In studies of playground games, children who begin coming to the playground learn the games already being played there, and when they leave, newcomers have the same access.[25] There is every reason to assume that students pick up the customs of college life from other students who are already there when they arrive. It is therefore important not to lose the sociality of four-year colleges by taking a false lesson that everything can just as well be moved online simply because that will preserve the kernel of knowledge and skills. It may preserve the kernel, but at the cost of the apparent chaff from a professorial perspective, which may be the heart of college experience from a student perspective.

New Lessons Learned for Now and After COVID-19

Something could be done about the usual knowledge and skills imparted in higher education, which despite the outreach of public intellectuals and the drive of progressive scholars to develop relevant material, tend to remain pretty much as they have always been. Pandemic disruptions have not tarnished the memory, and many long to go back. However, these disruptions, combined with how they have affected our students and what they think about them, could inspire real curricula change in the humanities and liberal arts, particularly philosophy. The political views of college students who organize, protest, and demonstrate have coalesced peer-to-peer from in-person contact and social media transmission.

Insofar as college students were a large part of the twenty-six million George Floyd/Black Lives Matter 2020 protests, these views developed autonomously and in some degree of isolation and even alienation from professors and administrators, especially since colleges were closed down by the time these protests began. For instance, while the exact number of college students who participated in these protests appears not to have been calculated, *Forbes* relates these protests to the 1960s civil rights demonstrations and lists a number of factors sparking young adult (i.e., ages eighteen through twenty-four) activism at the present time: the Black Lives Matter movement already has broad support; reactions against racist symbols in building names and monuments on campuses; the unpopularity of President Trump among this group; 93 percent of college students recently polled said that charging the same tuition for online as in-person education is unjust; the use of social media magnifies calls to protest.[26] *Forbes* is a global media company, covering business, technology, social trends, the economy, and investing—in essence, a gyroscope for the mainstream. So, one could add a sixth factor to the likelihood of ongoing student protest—namely, that it will be expected. And, of course, there is the seventh factor of absence from campus resulting in pent-up energy in need of an outlet. If the George Floyd/Black Lives Matter protests were largely driven by "furloughed" college students (as the mainstream believes), then the force of student political and cultural opinion has finally come into its own in the United States. This is one of the most important effects of COVID-19.

The college students of today are the local and national leaders and teachers of tomorrow. Their own future roles as leaders and teachers develop haphazardly, without foundation, structure, or intellectual resources from institutions of higher education. The issue here is not whether more surveillance or control would be desirable. Rather, the inchoate politics of college youth could bring everyone closer to a resource-rich, egalitarian, and benevolent society if traditional curricula were less removed from their nurturance.

John Dewey provided a beginning for how to think about such educational innovation, in philosophical projects that legitimately attend to education as an integral part of the process of doing philosophy. Dewey was aware of the importance of new ideas, problem solving, and cultural plurality as integral parts of democratic education or educated democracy. He may have been talking about the current (or any) generation of college students when he wrote:

> There will be almost a revolution in school education when study and learning are treated not as acquisition of what others know but as development of capital to be invested in eager alertness in observing and judging the conditions under which one lives. Yet until this happens, we shall be ill-prepared to deal with a world whose outstanding trait is change.[27]

We also can credit Dewey with the core idea of multicultural education as a need to accept students as already imbedded in communities outside of the classroom. In "Ethical Principles Underlying Education," he wrote, "The school cannot be a preparation for social life excepting as it reproduces, within itself, the typical conditions of social life."[28] If students, on all levels of the educational system, bring their community cultures with them and, as Dewey insisted, the interests of these cultures are entitled to be part of the educational system, this in itself is reason to have curricula constructed by teachers from, and with content concerning, those groups in society from which students come. It is inadequate to present students from diverse backgrounds with curricula content constructed by and about members of a privileged race and gender—that is, by and about white men. We already know this, but something has for a long time been missing in its implementation.

The college student population at four-year institutions lives in a bubble of college culture. A truly multicultural higher education would need to be fully integrated regarding race, ethnicity, and family income and wealth. This means that four-year institutions will need to become cheaper to attend, that new four-year institutions will need to be created, or that financial aid for college tuition will require more government assistance. And while we envision something like universal college education, returning again to Dewey, there will need to be better bridges between life on campus and life in the real world.

An essential part of the connection of higher education to the real world is the simple matter of access. Scott Galloway, who teaches at the NYU Stern School of Business, has predicted that COVID-19 will accelerate recent trends in access to higher education. The past forty years have seen higher endowments and greater exclusivity for Harvard, Yale, Stanford, and their cohort. Public and state schools remain good value and certification at low cost, but middle-tier colleges and universities have been raising tuition, without increasing value. In coping with the pandemic and thriving beyond it, top-tier universities will be able to ride out drops in tuition by remaining fully online, while at the same time preserving the exclusivity of their brands; inexpensive public schools will lose little in tuition or admissions by online teaching. But middle-tier schools have been going through contortions to support on-campus attendance in order to preserve tuition revenues. Measures have included frequent testing, stricter enforcement of social distancing, predictions of outbreaks that include analysis of sewage from dorms (if SARS-CoV-2 is detected in a batch of fecal matter, the entire dorm can be tested), and apps that allow for contact tracing.[29] Galloway suggests that unless this middle tier adapts with better and smarter use of technology, which makes their tuition affordable to middle-class families, many institutions will go under.[30]

The COVID-19 pandemic has resulted in cuts to all sources of funding for higher education, from Harvard University to little-known regional institutions. On the eve of the 2020 presidential election, it was estimated that lost revenue thus far totaled $120 billion (or over 20 percent of the higher education budget). In order to cope, there have been cuts to majors and programs in the social sciences and humanities, as well as furloughs, early retirements, and terminations of full-time, unionized faculty.[31]

The refuge dimension of college attendance and scholarly work is part of its attraction for many, and the life of the mind has its own consolations and justifications, especially in a secular society. However, here we should carry on with what Dewey left out of his vision of philosophy—as the philosophy of education pertaining to all fields— and that's the content of what philosophers study and teach. Regardless of how relevant they may strive to be, that present content remains woefully removed from reality.

As practitioners of an ancient discipline, philosophers philosophize philosophy. That is, they write, speak, and think—almost exclusively— about the philosophical work of other philosophers. Nietzsche undoubtedly had something like this in mind when he referred to the occupational practice of taxidermy (in the third epigraph to this chapter). But it is worse than that. It would be like that if philosophers talked about real life and real politics in the recent past—that is, if they philosophized the unphilosophical of ten or twenty years ago. But they do not do that. They do not even attend to history or biography in treatments of revered idols from centuries or millennia past.

What is needed is a philosophy of the unphilosophical, as it happens. I have tried to do this in the present text and previous publications— indeed, in most of my work. I cannot defend it as philosophy except to say that I continue to be employed to teach in a department of philosophy in an institution of higher education and my work is published as philosophy. For a troubled time, I encourage others in philosophy and other fields in the humanities and liberal arts to turn their scholarship and pedagogy toward what is happening, what is in the news, at the time they are working. If enough of us are committed to doing this, then some of the students in our four-year colleges will learn durable skills for considering the nature of the world in which they will lead and teach.

This would be attention to change, as Dewey said. It would be attention to what is urgent for protecting life, both human and environmental, in the present and for the future. If philosophers had a history of attending to the urgencies and emergencies of their own time, life on this planet would already be close to the utopias imagined by the most optimistic Panglossians. What other philosophers have written may be brought into such direct considerations to, as Locke put it, "enliven a busy scene," but the main source for immediate contemporary philosophy ought to be journalism, because journalism provides the primary record for what will become history.

Finally, the changes indicated by COVID-19 are not all aspirational on behalf of the adolescent and young adult denizens of leafy campuses, as the foregoing suggestions about higher education might suggest. The social aspects of COVID-19 effects on primary education have and will continue to shape the lives of mothers in ways that speak to theoretical feminist concerns and concrete lives. Coincidentally, the centennial of the Nineteenth Amendment occurred in the midst of back-to-school tensions in August 2020. The separation of life services from education in terms of knowledge and skills has not only an institutional side in terms of what educational institutions might be expected to provide but also real-life effects on the ability of women to work and participate in civic life. This is the child-care issue, already mentioned in chapter 4 as an ironic back-to-school push from those who may earlier have been ambivalent about women working outside of the home, but now know that they need them to restart the economy. Also, for decades, feminists have expressed concern about working women's "second shift" of child-care and domestic chores, following their work hours outside of the home. Few women with young children are immune to such responsibilities. In mid-July 2020, the gendered effect in the sciences was summed up in *Nature*:

> COVID-19 has not affected all scientists equally. A survey of principal investigators indicates that female scientists, those in the "bench sciences" and, especially, scientists with young children experienced a substantial decline in time devoted to research. This could have important short and longer-term effects on their careers, which institution leaders and funders need to address carefully.[32]

Twenty-four/seven, 365-day-a-year neighborhood child care and child minding would solve this problem, not only for working mothers during the pandemic but also in the new reality to follow. A US Census Bureau survey from July 16 to July 21 showed that about 31 percent of women with children at home, compared to 11.6 percent of men, were not working because of child-care duties.[33] A national child-care program would provide equity for this situation.

Before national child care is in effect, or for women who choose not to avail themselves of it, why has there been no initiative for national pay for housework and child care? A 2020 calculation by Salary.com put the wages of a homemaker with children and other domestic duties (including cooking, cleaning, chauffeuring) at $178,000, which would amount to trillions if all who did this work were paid.[34] However, the high price tag is too easily dismissed and can be viewed as a *reductio ad absurdum*. More modest financial support for unpaid domestic work and child care remains a live issue.

Altogether, the Women's Suffrage Centennial is a reminder of women's untapped political power. There are more women than ever holding political office or running for it, on all levels. This points not only to the importance of women voting but also to the need that women follow through after they vote. Such follow-through includes holding the candidates they voted for accountable and speaking out against less progressive candidates who win. This kind of informed and activist voting requires knowledge of relevant issues that affect not only women or mothers and children but everyone. Women have been designated the universal caregivers, and since so many have embraced that role, what is good for women is likely to also be good for those of other genders.[35] This need for active and politically activist voting requires both knowledge and skill, verified factual information, and tried-and-true practical methods, such as the ability to organize and demonstrate.

So here we come back to the importance of education, as well as the importance of civic participation, not only during the present pandemic but always in a democracy. Indeed, one of the traditional virtues of formal education has been its encouragement of civic responsibilities, of citizen building. Since the fall of 1988, the number of female students in higher education programs has exceeded the number of male students—56 to 44 percent.[36] There is, therefore, every reason to believe that women in the United States are already poised to fulfill full citizen duties. The disproportionate pressures on women during the time of COVID-19 have revealed structural fault lines that they may finally be willing, as well as able, to stabilize.

7

ECONOMY

"There are no nations, there are no peoples. There is only one who-
listic system of systems, one vast, interwoven, interacting, multivari-
ant, multinational domain of dollars. It is the international system of
currency which determines the totality of life on this planet. That is
the natural order of things today."
                          —Ned Beatty as Arthur Jensen in *Network*[1]

"Now money is necessary to all sorts of Men, as serving both for
Counters and for Pledges, and so carrying with it even Reckoning,
and Security, that he, that receives it, shall have the same Value for it
again, of other things that he wants, whenever he pleases. The one of
these it does by its Stamp and Denomination; the other by its intrinsick Value, which is its Quantity. The intrinsick Value of Silver and
Gold used in Commerce is nothing but their quantity."
                                              —John Locke, 1691[2]

Ever since the first quarantines and shutdowns during COVID-19, the
American public has been told that we are on the brink of the worst
recession or depression since 1929. Unemployment was at all-time
highs and the general economy had contracted according to leading
indicators. But home sale prices held firm, and after an initial dip in
February 2020, the stock market quickly recovered and, with slight
turbulence, remained close to its all-time highs by fall 2020, with a total
capitalization of about $35.5 trillion.[3] Earlier tax cuts and the Coronavi-
rus Aid, Relief, and Economic Security (CARES) Act were a positive
boon to the wealthiest Americans and largest corporations, while relief

was provided to unemployed or furloughed workers as well.[4] The wealth at the top did not trickle down, so the main question is whether the losses to unemployed households and small business closures will "trickle up." Will Main Street bring down Wall Street in a way that will spiral into more losses for Main Street, as pension funds are depleted and companies contract when their stock prices decline and workers are laid off? That is, will COVID-19 result in a (more) bifurcated economy between rich and poor, or will the entire system tank? This is not an idle question, because record-high unemployment has not motivated Republicans, who are generally loyal to the interests of big corporations, to open government coffers to aid those people and small businesses who are suffering the most. The bifurcated economy is so far mainly a problem for those in the bottom third.

As the epigraphs to this chapter indicate, the dominant representation of the economy is a universe of US dollars. Quite simply, dollars are the keys that open the doors to the material (and some immaterial) goods of human life. Without dollars or credit based on future dollars, there is no food, no clothing, no dwelling place. Dollars are no longer tied to anything with intrinsic value, such as gold or silver, but they have their own intrinsic value in their pure quantities. More money is more value. John Locke realized in the late 1600s that money itself provides its own intrinsic value based on its amount. He wrote about money in a system that tied the value of money to gold and silver—money in seventeenth-century England literally was gold and silver—and the more gold and silver was at the disposal of an individual or a nation, the more money it had.[5] In varied phases after Locke's day, actual currency ceased to be made of precious metals and became paper that represented quantities of gold or silver, and then the paper came to represent nothing except the backing of the national government. Today, not only does our money float free of anything of intrinsic value, but most of it is paid out, collected, and stored as marks in parts of "cyberspace."

Electronic entries in US dollars—the world currency, for all practical purposes—has nothing officially "backing it up" except the US government and, in principle, the totality of the US material economy, the components of which have prices or worth in dollars. The connection of money to the material economy is the ability to buy parts of it— that is, transfer the ownership or use of physical things and services in return for differences in electronic entries. The US government determines amounts of dollars in circulation, and what they can buy are either more dollars if they are invested (money making money) or the goods and services in the material economy. This fiat nature of dollars is brought home by Robert Hockett and Aaron James in *Money from Nothing: Or, Why We Should Stop Worrying about Debt and Learn to Love the Federal Reserve*. Hockett and James argue for the fiscal soundness of increased federal spending on programs for public works and measures to lessen income inequality, claiming that inflation can be managed and deficits viewed as a segment of public wealth, because deficits are money the people owe to themselves.[6] The fiat nature of dollars has been acknowledged for a long time, but it has not, in political terms, been connected to safety-net or other transfer programs. For instance, progressives typically approach income inequality as a matter of raising taxes on corporations and rich individuals, and conservatives are averse to government deficits. Neither side takes seriously the idea that money can be created out of nothing. If money can be created out of nothing, there is no reason to raise taxes on anyone, and deficits, as money owed by the government, can be bought out by creating more money.

As long as government maintains its authority and the real economy of what money can buy continues to function, deficits are an abstract problem. If this remains a concern for conservatives, it can be argued that a healthy real economy, with low unemployment, will result in greater productivity to balance out the deficit. Also, those employed will spend their earnings, providing further fuel for the real economy. If this reasoning is sound, then the ideology against deficit spending may be less economic than social. The concern about a government outspending its earnings (from taxes), which goes back to seventeenth-century mercantilism, may today reduce the concern that those who are not earning their livelihood should not receive government support, because they do not deserve it. Socially, this is a position about how those who are not poor ought to treat those who are poor. And such concern might rest on a moral attitude to the effect that those who have not earned their livelihood ought to be left as they are. Without government creation and use of fiat money to decrease injustice, the realities that are tied to dollars as presently allocated determine how human beings, except for those whose work is to manipulate, manage, or play with money, experience the material reality in their actual lives. When dollars are used as reasons not to do what would otherwise be just, the fiat nature of dollars means that cost cannot be accepted as a real barrier if there is a political will to create more dollars for a just or humanitarian cause.

But, of course, there are values apart from dollar costs, which are matters of moral, ideological, and political difference, and how such values affect the distribution of dollars is an important point of contention. This chapter begins with some facts and figures about the dollar economy in the United States. Next, there is a discussion regarding how COVID-19 has shown the inadequacy of thinking only in those dollar terms about both the economy and new opportunities for economic change. The situation of so-called essential workers is as much qualitative as monetary and deserves a separate section. Furthermore, the injustice of inequalities in the economy reintroduces the important role played by the police, in normal times as well as during the COVID-19 pandemic. The chapter ends with further considerations.

THE COVID-19 US ECONOMY

As stated in chapter 6, the gross national product (GNP), or total value of all goods and services or total national expenditure in the United States, is about $20 trillion. Included in this figure is income from abroad, so the more precise indicator of the dollar value in the US economy is the gross domestic product (GDP). There is also the gross national income (GNI), which is the sum of the value of goods and services produced by US Nationals, both at home and abroad. For our purposes, any of these three indicators are useful to give a sense of scale, because over the past few years, they have varied only by about half a trillion dollars—that is, from $20 trillion to $21 trillion:[7]

GNP = Consumption + Investment + Government Expenditure + Net exports (imports – exports) + net trade (exports – imports) from abroad

[or]

GNP = GDP + net trade from abroad[8]

And:

GNI = GNP + income from investments abroad[9]

It makes sense to take a look at the expense segments according to all three of these indicators. The sectors of the US GDP were as follows on December 7, 2019: agriculture = 0.9% (2017 est.), industry = 19.1% (2017 est.), services = 80% (2017 est.).[10] The twelve Global Industry Stock Classification stock market sectors look slightly different: Energy, Materials, Industrials, Consumer Discretionary, Consumer Staples, Health Care, Financials, Information Technology, Telecommunication Services, Utilities, and Real Estate.[11]

At different times, COVID-19 has closed down all but essential services (e.g., food processing and deliveries, utilities, transportation, policing), which require face-to-face contact. Whatever can be done online has become digital so that physical retail stores, transportation (especially air travel and related hospitality services), mass entertainment, cultural venues and events, and sports events have been closed or reopened on restricted bases. No forms of education resemble their pre-pandemic forms. The immediate result of the pandemic has thus been severe economic loss for many employed in such "nonessential" sectors. Only those who can work without coming into physical contact or proximity with others have not suffered economically. By the summer of 2020, the US Bureau of Economic Analysis displayed the chart shown on the next page (figure 7.1), summarizing the first nine months (three quarters) of COVID-19 in the United States economy.

The US GDP decreased 5 percent at an annual rate in the first quarter of 2020 and 31.7 percent in the second quarter.[12] In the third quarter, just before the election, the GDP grew 7.4 percent from the second quarter, continuing an upswing with an uncertain future. The overall 2020 economy was thereby projected to be 4–5 percent smaller than before the pandemic.[13] While this contraction is not of either depression or even severe recession proportions, it has been devastating for nonessential workers whose work requires proximity or contact with others.

When the stock market cratered in early March 2020 and almost fifteen million were unemployed, the Republican administration and Congress crafted the $3 trillion stimulus package, which, together with reopenings, brought unemployment down. Some businesses were able

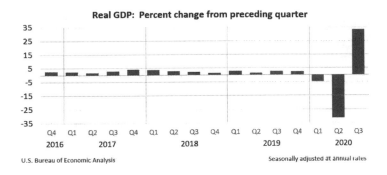

Figure 7.1.   Bureau of Economic Advancement GDP Report. Released November 25, 2020. (*Source:* https://www.bea.gov/news/glance)

to get loans, and unemployed individuals received stimulus checks of $600 a week. A moratorium on foreclosures and evictions became widespread. The financial markets stabilized and began making new highs in late August 2020. However, over the summer, another round of stimulus payments had stalled between the US House of Representatives and Senate. President Trump issued an executive order that included $300 federal payments to those unemployed, but it was not implemented, because Congress controls the purse.[14] In August 2020, the unemployment rate was down to 8.4 percent with 14.6 million unemployed. This was still more than double the February 2020 rate of 3.5 percent with 6.8 million unemployed.[15] By the end of the third quarter, the unemployment rate was 7.9 percent compared to about 3.8 percent the year before.[16]

Many think that Wall Street predicts Main Street by about six or nine months, because the stock prices of companies are based on their future earnings, and future earnings depend on real transactions involving companies' goods and services (although price-earnings ratios themselves vary with overall market sentiment, trending higher in bull markets and lower in bear markets).[17] But generally, in this case, the falling unemployment rate was predicted by stock market strength throughout the pandemic. Going into the fall of 2020, it was unknown how the dollar-calculated US economy would fare, were the pandemic to worsen. And it was of course unknown who would win the election.

What was widely known by then is that the US economy was already intensely politicized, with Democrats emphasizing contraction and unemployment and Republicans insisting that recovery to previous highs had been in process for months. It should be understood that stock market newsletters and magazines are generally nonpolitical. For instance, after earlier forecasts of the effects of the 2020 election results on the financial markets, the financial news publication *Barron's* concluded in mid-September that markets would be "rocky" no matter who won.[18] In any event, analyses and recommendations of financial markets have traditionally been geared to the quality of investments in terms solely of their profitability. Nonetheless, in early October 2020, *Barron's* noted that more fiscal stimulus was positively anticipated as the economic recovery faltered.[19]

It will be impossible to fully describe the COVID-19 US economy until the pandemic is past or under control to a high degree of probability. On November 10, 2020, the CDC announced that only a 15 percent increase in mask wearing could save a loss of $1 trillion. In addition, hopes placed on an effective vaccine and widely distributed antiviral medications will not be fulfilled until spring or summer of 2021.[20]

Essential Workers

Simultaneously with initial lockdowns and quarantines in the Northeast, and in other states that mitigated in the same way, the term "essential workers" sprang up. The idea seems to have been that some workers were too necessary for the continuation of even limited social and economic functioning to be furloughed or fired. And because their work involves doing something physical outside of their homes, they cannot work from home. Essential workers include police officers, fire responders, medical first responders, doctors, nurses, delivery people, grocery and pharmacy workers, defense workers, janitors, and scores of other kinds of workers in utilities, transportation, agriculture, and child care.[21] There were federal and state guidelines (and, in some places, no guidelines) for their employment during the pandemic. Many have been obligated to report for work, and except for doctors, the physical work performed by essential workers is not high-status work in US society. (Doctors are a complex group because it is difficult to imagine them refusing to show up because of concerns about their fatigue or personal safety; this makes it is easy to presume that they have a calling or strong sense of occupational obligation. But much of what many of them do is physical work in very close contact with patients.)

According to the data from 2017–2018 that was posted in May 2020, essential workers comprise 70 percent of the normal, pre-COVID-19 US labor force and earn an average hourly wage of $27.25. Not all essential workers—for instance, those employed by airlines—have continued to be employed during the pandemic. The total workforce of essential workers is composed of slightly more men than women.

Frontline workers, who overlap with essential workers, have direct contact with members of the public. They disproportionately have socioeconomically disadvantaged backgrounds and earn an hourly average of $21.85. About 80 percent of frontline workers are in essential industries (and are thereby part of the 70 percent of the workforce constituted by essential workers), and they comprise about one-third of the total labor force. They are mostly male, include a higher proportion of racial and ethnic minorities than the general workforce, and are less educated.[22]

Overall, essential workers and frontline workers, in particular, do physical work that brings them into contact with other people so that they are more vulnerable to COVID-19 contagion than those who work at home. But the labels can be misleading, because they leave out contact with other workers; for example, essential workers (who are not frontline workers) employed in meat-processing plants have had high rates of infection as a result of long hours in cramped conditions in cold temperatures.[23] Generally, physical work of the kind done by most frontline and other essential workers does not require a college degree or pay solid middle-class wages. Many of these workers do not have adequate health insurance or paid sick leave. Many have been required to work without adequate PPE or the ability to practice social distancing at their jobs.

It is a sociological truism that the so-called wealth curve rises to better health as income rises. Along with greater wealth comes more education, mainly a college degree. The assumed causal sequence is that wealthier families send their children to college, and their children in turn have higher incomes and, with that, nonphysical employment. That is, college graduates are not likely to be low-paid essential or frontline workers in the present pandemic.

However, recent analyses suggest that health is more directly an effect of higher education rather than simply an intersection with wealth or income. John Mirowsky and Catherine E. Ross point out that although wealth or income may buy more interactions with the health-care system, good health is not highly correlated with doctor or hospital visits, but rather the reverse. That is, people who are healthy have less need of the health-care system. So what makes them healthy? More education! This hypothesis is backed up with data showing that if income is held constant, education is positively correlated with good health. Mirowsky and Ross hypothesize that education increases autonomy in choosing interesting work, which reduces stress-caused illness. Education also gives people the willingness to acquire knowledge about healthy lifestyle choices and habits.[24]

Mirowsky and Ross's findings suggest further interesting aspects of essential work during COVID-19 in the United States. Not only are low-paid essential and frontline workers employed in jobs that they might not choose if they had more advanced educational certification, but their lack of formal education has also directly endangered their health in the jobs they are presently obligated to perform. Many of these jobs may already have higher risks of injury, as well as fatigue, but their intersection with COVID-19 has made them extremely hazardous.

Observers and political leaders have not lost sight of the necessity for essential and frontline work in a pandemic. Without it, others would be unable to quarantine, practice social distancing, or get health care. The CARES Act temporarily supplemented unemployment payments with $600 a week. There has been concern that this benefit may leave some better off economically if unemployed than employed.[25] Partly as an incentive to work, hazard pay has been proposed for frontline workers. Such hazard pay would also compensate them for the risk of contracting COVID-19 by continuing to work. In addition, many would receive support for child care, paid sick leave, health insurance, and death benefits to the families of those who have died from the virus. Legislation has passed for the Heroes Act along these lines in the US House of Representatives, but it has stalled in the US Senate.[26]

The second quarter 2020 jobs report indicated that the bottom third in income have suffered the most unemployment. Unemployment for longer than six months is taken to be an indication of permanent withdrawal from the workforce. Analysts have expressed further concern that many jobs lost in the service and retail sectors may have been permanently obliterated by the pandemic.[27]

Assuming the Heroes Act or something like it does eventually clear the Senate, it will have historical precedent. The so-called Spanish Flu also had designations of essential workers. This work was revalued over the course of the pandemic, with the eventual result of higher wages and, according to some historians, the momentum for the labor movement. Well before the Spanish Flu, medieval outbreaks of bubonic plague in Europe are credited with similar effects, such as putting an end to feudalism, as well as raising wages. But, of course, it's too soon to tell whether this history will repeat itself on the other side of COVID-19 in the United States, given the high probability of sluggish economic growth and the possibility of social disruption.[28]

The US economy has been politicized in two main ways. The first is the role of government in the dollar or financial economy, which is vast; the second is the influence of political party ideology on government economic programs, which are about reality as well as dollars. On the government side, neoliberalism or neoconservatism has been been the dominant political ideology since the Ronald Reagan administration (1981–1989), encompassing free trade, low taxes, deregulation, privatization, and balanced government budgets. While free trade and balanced budgets are flexible goals for Republican administrations, privatization and deregulation have made substantial inroads against safety-net and support programs for poor working people and others who can be assisted only through federal government action. This process has produced a chasm between the very wealthy and everyone else, as national wealth in dollars has been transferred upward.[29] The Democratic and Republican national conventions of 2020 also expressed a chasm. Democrats emphasized the ravages of COVID-19, while Republicans all but ignored it. Democrats referred to programs that would support the poor and unemployed, create infrastructure and jobs to address climate change, and effectively address the pandemic, as a precondition for economic recovery. But Republicans emphasized a booming stock market, high real estate sales, and a rise in employment from spring 2020 levels.[30]

Politicians do not need to delve deeply into ideology or political theory in order to attract votes, because appealing public policy proposals are sufficient to spell out who will benefit from their party platforms. However, cultural observers and political theorists work from more developed ideas and ideals regarding the economy, especially given the opportunity for creative thought provided by a disaster. This is not restricted to individual creativity, but extends in applications of a characteristic of extreme change as an opportunity to push forward predeveloped agendas. For instance, Naomi Klein in *The Shock Doctrine* highlights aggressive right-wing uses of capitalist tools for further concentrating wealth behind the screen of disaster. In that book and subsequent articles, Klein showed how the same corporations that benefited from the Iraq War were able to increase their wealth in the aftermath of Hurricane Katrina.[31]

In late March 2020, Klein (along with documentary filmmaker and writer Astra Taylor and Keeanga-Yamahtta Taylor, professor of African American Studies at Princeton University) conducted a virtual teach-in that drew a global audience of 14,000.[32] Their thesis stood on its head the customary idea that COVID-19 had disrupted normal life. According to these thinkers, the capitalistic economic system was already economically unjust against those who came to be seen as essential workers, as well as women and the poor. They therefore claimed that well before the pandemic, capitalism was disproportionately killing these people. Because they considered unjust economic distribution detrimental to life, Klein and her colleagues offered a foundation for economic justice programs during the pandemic, which were more than a response to the pandemic.

THE POLICE, PROPERTY, AND POVERTY

In a *New Yorker* magazine essay, Keeanga-Yamahtta Taylor analyzed the economic issues related to the George Floyd/Black Lives Matter protests as having included centuries of systematic economic oppression of African Americans. According to Taylor, proposals to "defund" the police, who receive the lion's share of budgets in US cities with high black populations, would be a way to dislodge the racial oppression practiced throughout US society, because the police are on the front lines for keeping that injustice in place. Taylor suggests that for real change, the unjust prison system would need to be dismantled, nationwide child care would be required, and a high-quality educational system would need to be accessible for all, as would sick leave and afford-able or free medical care.[33] Taylor's focus is on African Americans who suffer from social injustice as the result of economic injustice, and the present George Floyd/Black Lives Matter protests bring us back to the issue of police conduct. Taylor quotes from "We Charge Genocide," a petition submitted to the United Nations in 1951 by activists in Harlem:

> Once the classic method of lynching was the rope. Now it is the policeman's bullet. To many an American the police are the govern-ment, certainly its most visible representative. We submit that the evidence suggests that the killing of Negroes has become police poli-cy in the United States and that police policy is the most practical expression of government policy.[34]

It is very important that, for many Americans, the police are the government. One of the chief duties of the government is to protect private property. Normal police behavior, without egregious miscon-duct, is intimidating to those who are socially disadvantaged—that is, to those who are not deemed worthy of protection because they do not own property (e.g., African Americans). When African Americans protest violently against egregious police injustice, some private proper-ty destruction occurs, which may be a symbolic attack on the institution of private property from which many are excluded. This situation in turn leads to further violence and calls for violence against violent pro-testers to back up the police. Short of full-out revolution, the police, who do represent the government, must prevail.

The dynamic of property destruction by protesters symbolizes an important connection to the economy, especially during the COVID-19 pandemic. The US economy is normally unequal, and that inequality, insofar as it disproportionately affects minorities, is unjust. COVID-19 has revealed that injustice, both economically and medically. Even nor-mal police misconduct can be seen in a new light as oppressive and egregious misconduct that is unacceptably oppressive. But again, as Taylor points out, the normal racist oppression of African Americans by police is connected to the systematic economic inequality as an attempt to protect that inequality.

African Americans are not the only group that suffers from econom-ic injustice, despite their disproportionate presence among the incar-cerated, ill, exploited, and undereducated. Latinx and Native Americans also experience disproportionate inequalities. Nevertheless, it is white Americans who have the largest absolute (not relative) numbers in these disadvantaged groups. Therefore, the full implication of Taylor's analysis is not so much to propose a remedy for racism, institutional or otherwise, but a remedy for all underlying social ills that are related to economic inequality. Taylor assumes that racism is a symptom of this underlying economic inequality, or that the economic inequality is already racist. But the economic inequality extends well beyond race, as figure 7.2 (for 2018) shows.

Poverty decreased to 11.8 percent of the population in 2018, from 12.3 percent in 2017. However, the US poverty rate has been stable over the past thirty years, with an average of 13.4 percent.[35] Poverty figures as a result of COVID-19 are yet to be compiled, but insofar as people of color have been disproportionately unemployed and ill, the racial poverty differences are likely to increase, as is overall poverty.

	All Americans In Category (Millions)	Americans In Poverty (Millions)	Poverty Rate
White, not Hispanic	194.6	14.2	7.3%
Black	43.0	8.1	18.8%
Asian	19.9	1.5	7.4%
Hispanic, any race	60.6	9.5	15.8%

Figure 7.2.   Federal Safety Net, US Poverty Statistics from US Census Bureau. Released September 2020. (*Source:* http://federalsafetynet.com/us-poverty-statistics.html)

A total, nondiscriminatory federal remedy for poverty in the United States, affecting the 38.1 million Americans who are poor, would appear to be a socialistic remedy, at least. And that trajectory has had famous theoretical advocates, ever since Karl Marx. Thomas Piketty's 2014 *Capital in the Twenty-First Century* explains persisting inequalities in wealth in terms of the ability of those already rich to passively accumulate capital through real estate investments, which is not matched by increases in total national wealth. Piketty therefore advocates a progressive tax on wealth.[36] In his 2020 *Pandemic!*, Slavoj Žižek explicitly advocates communism, because he believes that its central organization offers the only way for nations to emerge from COVID-19.[37] However, if government economic policy is presented without ideology, a mixed economy (part capitalistic and part safety net) could be reaffirmed insofar as it is already instituted.[38] That is, while the United States has a capitalist market economy, it also has guaranteed entitlements such as Social Security, Medicare, Medicaid, and varied fluctuaring aid programs for the poor, including the Affordable Care Act.

FURTHER CONSIDERATIONS

It is sobering to consider the US economy as an engine for the unequal distribution of wealth and disadvantage. This perspective suggests that racism and xenophobia are indeed the tip of the iceberg of money. The question raised is this: How much dollar inequality is just in a democracy if the necessary goods of food, shelter, clothing, freedom, medical care, and knowledge are all dependent on dollars? Another way of posing this question is whether access to the necessary goods is a human right that should be protected in a democracy. If the United States is a democracy, is this a decision that can be decided by vote—in the current case, voting for a presidential candidate who is likely to view access to the necessary goods as rights, versus one who does not? By contrast, would the increase in federal government size and strength required to implement programs that redistributed wealth in themselves constrict democracy and the autonomy of those subscribed in such programs?

Disaster magnifies inequalities in dramatic ways and provides opportunities to propose structural changes. Such changes would be sound preparation for the next disaster, but their advocates usually have long-standing prior ideological commitments that motivate economic justice: abiding faith in strong government as a benevolent institution, and ideas of justice that include basic economic security. These commitments are of course opposed by those who valorize weak government with free markets and individual responsibility. Again, if the ideologies can be pushed aside and problems viewed practically, on the level of public policy, it might be possible to work around the ideological impasse by coming up with less contentious framing of public policy.

For instance, in international development discourse, disaster *mitigation* is often proposed as a way to both avoid the worst of future disasters and create better infrastructure in poor nations.[39] Poor communities in the United States, which have suffered most from COVID-19, could receive similar kinds of support that would make them more resilient in future disasters, as well as build up their resources for normal times. This would involve spending on K–12 education, as well as child care, and making sources of nutritious food and affordable medical care more accessible. Another nonideological concept is *sustainability*, often employed in the context of climate change.[40] Sustainable practices do not exhaust the resources they use, and sustainable jobs would not exhaust the human resources they require. In terms of the kinds of economic disparities experienced in COVID-19, job training ought to be sustainable. Sustainable job training would be not simply geared to specific jobs but to kinds of jobs across industries, so that skills become transferable if a person loses a particular job. The ideas of both mitigation and sustainability can be presented wholly in terms of programs that accomplish specific goals, to bypass traditional ideological conflict. This would not be a move in rhetoric or propaganda, because, in reality, ideologies float free of specific problems and are mainly used as tools for political persuasion and manipulation.

8

MEDIA

"Then [Barack Obama] pretended to sit back and press the remote to turn on a television. 'That's not activism. That's not bringing about change,' he said. 'If all you're doing is casting stones, you're probably not going to get that far. That's easy to do.'"
—Emily S. Rueb and Derrick Bryson Taylor, *New York Times*, reporting on the Obama Foundation Summit, October 29, 2019[1]

"Keep your friends close, but your enemies closer."
—*The Godfather: Part II* (1974)[2]

A major theme of this book has been the distinction and contrast between rhetoric and reality in our time. Rhetoric has been easy enough to identify as mere discourse. Reality is, presumably, that which exists outside of rhetoric—it is primary, fundamental, ultimate—although this does not mean that it can be experienced without description. Roughly speaking, true descriptions seem to justify themselves. However, so does rhetoric. The difference is that true descriptions are linked to something outside of themselves, in orderly ways that are missing in rhetoric. Of course, the emphasis here is on truth, but truth can tilt toward what it is that people believe, especially in disaster, as E. L. Quarantelli defined it (see chapter 1). That is, if enough people react to an event as though it is a disaster, then the event is a disaster. But not everything believed in such a reaction is necessarily true, because there can be mass panics that are not based on real dangers. Also, there may be intense disagreement about the nature of a danger (for instance, between scientifically oriented groups who believe that vaccinations contribute to better health and those who believe that vaccinations are a threat to health and the cause of new diseases). For example, some believe there are causal links between COVID-19 and earlier immunizations against diseases (as will be discussed in chapter 9).

Because reality is primary and fundamental, there is a preference for true beliefs about our current disaster, not only because of an age-old fealty to and love of truth but also for the practical reason that true descriptions will enable actions that are more likely to have desired consequences than false ones, and predictions based on true descriptions are more reliable for preparing for the future than those based on falsehood.

Rhetoric is shared, and many now live within collective rhetoric or do not make the distinction between self-contained and true discourse. Doing that would require critical examination of the content of rhetoric in terms of its truth—that is, its connection to reality. It should not be surprising that in the absence of cohesive and coherent discourse from national leadership, truth, falsehood, rumor, and speculation coexist within society. A lot of energy is devoted to discourse about events. The rhetoric of this social dimension of public life becomes dominant over the content of shared beliefs. In the United States, this social, rhetorical dimension encompasses literal public speech and action that includes physical demonstration or protests, as well as private or semi-public expression via electronic social media. At the same time, opinion and discourse become more important leisure outlets, because pandemic mitigation measures have closed bars, restaurants, theaters, movie theaters, sports arenas, music concerts, and special interest and political meetings, among other collective activities. Vacation travel by plane, car, train, and ship has also been curtailed. There is still plenty of entertainment to stream or rent for home enjoyment, in addition to printed material, but the general eclipse of the outside world is a major contraction of outlets for communication and interaction outside of people's homes.

People not only do the same things in different ways and through different modalities but also engage in activities they have not done before and do more of what they can still do, with which they are already familiar. Some activities and forms of consumption, such as buying and preparing food and keeping apprised of what is happening, assume novel, heightened importance. But also, the rhetoric of loss about what cannot be done should be emphasized, because it has a real foundation in the absence of things and events.

Remaining informed through "getting the news" has taken on a new importance since the beginning of COVID-19. The news is now directly relevant to the circumstances of individual life, and getting it, as both a consumer and a citizen, has for many become an activity encroaching on or even supplanting entertainment, especially since COVID-19 mitigation has made it difficult for new movies and television shows, as well as sports events, to be produced. The news, consumed electronically, has become a primary connection to the outside world, which makes it more exciting, more engaging, and more important. This chapter therefore begins with a discussion of issues of facts, truth, and ethics involved in the presentation of news. We move from there to new questions about history that have emerged in the public issue of the symbolic role of statues and monuments, concluding with considerations of social media, specifically "cancel culture."

NEWS

It has been recognized since World War II that journalism—our collective source of information about what is going on in the world, and the primary record for history—is some mixture of facts and opinion. The best journalism is supposed to be fact-based. The opinions it conveys and does not merely report, even though they are identified as opinions, should also be fact-based. The *New York Times* is described by *Encyclopedia Britannica* as follows:

> The *New York Times*, morning daily newspaper published in New York City, long the newspaper of record in the United States and one of the world's great newspapers. Its strength is in its editorial excellence; it has never been the largest newspaper in terms of circulation. [3]

One would expect the *New York Times* to avoid blurring lines between falsehood and truth, especially in providing a platform for and not merely reporting opinions. A recent instance of its apparent failure to do that and the steps it took to self-correct are interesting in this regard. On July 3, 2020, the *New York Times* published the following op-ed by Senator Tom Cotton from Arkansas:

> Opinion: Tom Cotton: Send in the Troops / The Nation Must Restore Order. The Military Stands Ready.

> This week, rioters have plunged many American cities into anarchy, recalling the widespread violence of the 1960s.

> New York City suffered the worst of the riots Monday night, as Mayor Bill de Blasio stood by while Midtown Manhattan descended into lawlessness. Bands of looters roved the streets, smashing and emptying hundreds of businesses. Some even drove exotic cars; the riots were carnivals for the thrill-seeking rich as well as other criminal elements.

> Outnumbered police officers, encumbered by feckless politicians, bore the brunt of the violence. In New York State, rioters ran over officers with cars on at least three occasions. In Las Vegas, an officer is in "grave" condition after being shot in the head by a rioter. In St. Louis, four police officers were shot as they attempted to disperse a mob throwing bricks and dumping gasoline; in a separate incident, a 77-year-old retired police captain was shot to death as he tried to stop looters from ransacking a pawnshop. This is "somebody's granddaddy," a bystander screamed at the scene.

> Some elites have excused this orgy of violence in the spirit of radical chic, calling it an understandable response to the wrongful death of George Floyd. Those excuses are built on a revolting moral equivalence of rioters and looters to peaceful, law-abiding protesters. A majority who seek to protest peacefully shouldn't be confused with bands of miscreants.

There was an immediate response from *New York Times* readers and staff members, who pointed out factual inaccuracies in Cotton's op-ed and objected to its overall fascist or totalitarian ideological tone.[4] Cotton's article was subsequently published online with this statement above it:

> Editors' Note, June 5, 2020:

> After publication, this essay met strong criticism from many readers (and many *Times* colleagues), prompting editors to review the piece

and the editing process. Based on that review, we have concluded that the essay fell short of our standards and should not have been published.

The basic arguments advanced by Senator Cotton—however objectionable people may find them—represent a newsworthy part of the current debate. But given the life-and-death importance of the topic, the senator's influential position and the gravity of the steps he advocates, the essay should have undergone the highest level of scrutiny. Instead, the editing process was rushed and flawed, and senior editors were not sufficiently involved. While Senator Cotton and his staff cooperated fully in our editing process, the Op-Ed should have been subject to further substantial revisions—as is frequently the case with such essays—or rejected.

For example, the published piece presents as facts assertions about the role of "cadres of left-wing radicals like antifa"; in fact, those allegations have not been substantiated and have been widely questioned. Editors should have sought further corroboration of those assertions, or removed them from the piece. The assertion that police officers "bore the brunt" of the violence is an overstatement that should have been challenged. The essay also includes a reference to a "constitutional duty" that was intended as a paraphrase; it should not have been rendered as a quotation.

Beyond those factual questions, the tone of the essay in places is needlessly harsh and falls short of the thoughtful approach that advances useful debate. Editors should have offered suggestions to address those problems. The headline—which was written by the *Times*, not Senator Cotton—was incendiary and should not have been used.

Finally, we failed to offer appropriate additional context—either in the text or the presentation—that could have helped readers place Senator Cotton's views within a larger framework of debate.

The editor of the *New York Times* op-ed section resigned. The Cotton op-ed had not been this editor's first misjudgment. Since his hiring in 2016, he was responsible for printing an anti-Semitic cartoon in an international edition of the *New York Times* and allowing an alleged defamatory claim about former vice-presidential candidate Sarah Palin to be published. Nor was the *New York Times* unique in the kind of self-regulation precipitated by Cotton's op-ed. The main editor of the

Philadelphia Inquirer resigned after an article about the George Floyd protests appeared under the headline "Buildings Matter, Too."[5]

Most readers of sober and serious newspapers such as the *New York Times* and *Philadelphia Inquirer* rely on and trust them for true descriptions of reality. More than this, such sources have taken it upon themselves to maintain their probity and protect the appearance of it. This moral epistemological role of the most respectable and highly respected news publishers has been continually disparaged by President Trump and others in his administration who believe in "alternative facts" and, on that basis, refer to the *New York Times* as a source of "fake news."[6] Of course, the term *fake news* originated in descriptions of fabricated news stories on social media, but it has been weaponized by those who benefit from such real fake news. Still, the fake-news charge against them explains why newspapers of record would be sensitive about factual accuracy in general. However, the sensitivity displayed in the reasoning behind the editorial statement accompanying the subsequent posting of Cotton's op-ed, followed by the resignation of the op-ed editor, raises deeper questions that philosophers and other scholars of critical thinking might have greater flexibility in delving into than do newspaper publishers and editors. This issue involves the nature of the responsibility that newspaper editors and publishers have explicitly taken upon themselves since World War II.

In late 1943, Henry R. Luce, publisher of Time, Inc., sponsored a gathering of academics and policy makers in New York City, directed by Robert Hutchins, president of the University of Chicago, called the Commission on Freedom of the Press. The Commission met seventeen times over three years and interviewed over 50 witnesses, with an additional 225 interviews held by its staff. This work resulted in a short book, *A Free and Responsible Press.*[7] The Commission's purpose was to evaluate American journalism in answer to three questions: What society do we want? What do we have? How can journalism be used to get from the society we have to the society we want? There was concern about the spread of fascist ideas through US society, and members of the Commission were concerned about discord provoked by the press, which had resulted in "different worlds of fact and judgement."

The Hutchins Commission affirmed freedom of expression as the primary virtue of a democracy. They assumed that this political liberty is foundational to all others and the consumption of ideas is the lifeline of "civilized society." They identified five obligations of the press: provide a true, comprehensive, and intelligent account of the day's events; provide a forum for discussion of important viewpoints and interests in society; provide a "representative picture" of society and its groups; educate the public about community ideals; make information available to everybody. Competition for public attention, bias of publishers, and pressure from interest groups had so far prevented the fulfillment of these obligations,[8] rendering them ideals.

The reaction of the *New York Times* publishers to the Cotton op-ed does seem to share the subtext of responsible journalism that includes educating the public about community ideals, as well as reporting facts. However, the *New York Times* seems to have blurred the line between reporting facts on its own account and reporting the facts reported by those presenting "important viewpoints and interests in society." In this case, Cotton was presenting a viewpoint doubtless shared or at least aired by President Trump in his earlier militaristic response to the George Floyd/Black Lives Matter protests at the end of May 2020 (see chapters 2 and 3 for discussions of these events). In its reaction to Cotton's op-ed, the *New York Times* publishers seem to hold themselves responsible for the goodness or badness of the opinions expressed therein. So even if one agrees with the *New York Times*'s uber-editorial perspective on Cotton, one wonders why, instead of merely correcting Cotton's factual inaccuracy, more was not done to identify and attack Cotton's "world of fact and judgement"—that is, his ideology or the conceptual scheme within which his ideas made sense.

Cotton's conceptual scheme included the racial and political stereotyping of all George Floyd/Black Lives Matter protesters as dangerous, radical criminals, and its "facts" were hyperbolic exaggerations of what the real facts he purported to be reporting were. There are many social critics who could have argued against Cotton by identifying his conceptual scheme and its use of distorted facts. So, as an editorial matter, in overstepping its own responsibility, the *New York Times* failed to provide the necessary forum for discussion. We cannot assume that conceptual schemes we know are correct unless they are publicly made explicit and argued for, especially when they are under attack. The failure to understand this basic principle becomes grounds for pessimism, if not cynicism, about the best sources of news now available. This is not a matter of superficially presenting "both sides," which has justifiably been criticized when one side has more reason and logic, but rather allowing the arguments of both sides to be laid bare before the public. As John Stuart Mill, speaking of true, received opinions (or, in this context, "community ideals"), put it in *On Liberty*:

> Even if the received opinion be not only true, but the whole truth; unless it is suffered to be, and actually is, vigorously and earnestly contested, it will, by most of those who receive it, be held in the manner of a prejudice, with little comprehension or feeling of its rational grounds. [9]

In failing to allow for a wider, knock-down, drag-out discussion, the *New York Times*, in crudely "canceling" Cotton and his editor, stifled the freedom of expression that would have been exercised had others been afforded the opportunity to argue against him in place of mere fact checking. No one should believe that Cotton's perspective and misstatement of facts simply cease to exist if the newspaper of record summarily eschews them.

Another problem with the news of record is its attention span, the way that focal events crowd the crisis of the day before. In the days immediately following the November 3, 2020, election, COVID-19 was surging throughout the United States and cases of infection, as well as deaths, were recorded at unprecedented highs. The media put COVID-19 coverage on the back burner for several days. There are two aspects to this shift. The first is that the election was a valid distraction from the pandemic, which allowed the nation to concentrate on politics by voting and attending to media for the results. Except for the extension of mail-in voting and pandemic-mitigation measures in voting and vote counting, political participation in the 2020 election was not curtailed by the pandemic. The other aspect of the attention switch is that the election was widely believed to be mainly about how the federal government would address the pandemic. The election was thereby a higher-order causal factor for the future of pandemic response.

The news media of record are understood as presenting important news, but we do not know how the choice between featuring the election or the pandemic was made. The American public accepted the shift in media attention, which was temporary, because pandemic coverage quickly returned, to share the stage with Trump's objections to Biden's win. But besides its obligation to check facts, the media of record do not seem to perceive a need to justify what they consider primarily newsworthy.

THE WAR OVER THE STATUES

During the spring of 2020 amid the George Floyd protests, the Southern Poverty Law Center estimated that over 1,700 Confederate statues remained in public view throughout the United States. The arguments and efforts to remove them were well under way before the new George Floyd impetus during COVID-19. Those in favor of removal have focused on historical facts about the statues themselves, especially that those being honored were seeking to destroy the United States, as a Union, and that traitors ought not to be publicly honored.[10]

We should notice in this claim that, first, history is simplified to the Civil War being only about the retention of slavery. While that is not a bad simplification for progressive purposes, it does leave out issues of states' rights and how far some nineteenth-century Americans were willing to go to protect them, which has been progressively resurrected in our time, as discussed in chapter 2. That is, the precipitating issue of the Civil War was that Southern states seceded from the Union and they did so for a variety of economic reasons, in which slavery was a paramount consideration.[11] But as we have seen, the apparatus of states' rights in a federal system is both conceptually and practically distinct from what states want to use it to protect within their borders. However, in addition to the historical context of the subject of Confederate statues—that is, what they depict—the history of the statues themselves, as objects, is important.

Most of the Confederate monuments now facing removal were created not immediately after the Civil War, but rather during two periods in which African Americans were facing greater oppression while they were on the verge of greater civil liberty. During the Jim Crow era from the early 1890s to 1920, Confederate monuments were erected in Southern towns near government buildings at the time that voter suppression laws were passed. Others were dedicated or rededicated after the US Supreme Court ruling against school segregation in 1954. Bronze statues were prohibitively expensive, but the Monumental Bronze Company could sell zinc statues for under $500. Many private citizens, including the United Daughters of the Confederacy, were able to purchase statues that would be erected, displayed, and maintained on public land. [12] This history is aesthetically (as well as politically) tawdry, but other monuments with more legitimate origins have also been targets for removal, such as the Emancipation Memorial, as well as statues of lesser-known slave owners, racists, and Christopher Columbus. [13]

To discuss both the history of slavery and the Civil War and the history of the Confederate statues, in the context of those who seek their removal, plus the history of other candidates for removal, such as the Emancipation Memorial, is to enter a discourse that may be its own aim because it is an exchange of ideas about the relationship between symbols and reality. It is a discourse about historical events and history itself, brought to life by present events.

The Emancipation Memorial, also known as the "Freedman's Memorial" and the "Emancipation Group," is sited in Lincoln Park, in the Capitol Hill neighborhood of Washington, DC. It was designed by Thomas Ball and erected in 1876. Lincoln is iconographically depicted. His right hand rests on the Emancipation Proclamation that is on a pedestal, and his left arm is extended above a black man who kneels on one knee, naked to the waist, with his broken chain at Lincoln's feet. The statue of this former slave was a portrait of Archer Alexander, an emancipated slave. The funding for this memorial came from the wages of freed slaves. The memorial was proposed immediately after Lincoln's assassination, and Charlotte Scott, a former slave in Virginia, made the first contribution of $5 from her earnings. [14]

The word *Emancipation* appears on the base of the Emancipation Memorial. From its recent context of slavery, the Emancipation Memorial may have depicted a glorious historical moment. But even then, not all were happy with it. Soon after the monument was dedicated in 1876, Frederick Douglass focused on what the monument failed to record about political citizenship. He wrote:

> While the mere act of breaking the [N]egro's chains was the act of Abraham Lincoln . . . the act by which the negro was made a citizen of the United States and invested with the elective franchise was preeminently the act of President U. S. Grant, and this is nowhere seen in the Lincoln monument. . . . The negro here, though rising, is still on his knees and nude. What I want to see before I die is a monu-

ment representing the negro, not couchant on his knees like a four-footed animal, but erect on his feet like a man. There is room in Lincoln park for another monument, and I throw out this suggestion to the end that it may be taken up and acted upon.

More broadly, Douglass did not believe that any one monument could tell the whole truth.[15]

At this time, in the context of the George Floyd/Black Lives Matter movement, there is an urgent debate over whether the Emancipation Memorial should be removed—not because of unfulfilled promises to African Americans of full and equal citizenship, but rather because of its "optics": the monument shows a half-naked black man kneeling before a towering white man wearing formal clothes. A chain-link fence has been erected around the memorial, and in late June and early July 2020 police were guarding it. Critics have said that the depiction is degrading, because of the racial inequality plainly on view. Others, including African American activists, have insisted that Archer Alexander is in the process of rising, so that the memorial symbolizes aspiration. The memorial is on federal land, and if the mayor of Washington, DC, wanted to remove it, as other statues in cities throughout the country have been removed, she has no jurisdictional power to do that.[16] But if she could remove it, what would the reasons be? Lincoln did issue the Emancipation Proclamation, and many American slaves thereby became legally free. The statue was commissioned by freed slaves, and, when it continues to be defended by their descendants or cultural heirs, that historical fact is foremost.[17] But the optics are degrading in later contexts of racial egalitarianism.

Can the historical antiracism criticism motivating statue removal be reconciled with motivation based on how things look now? On the surface, it would seem that the optics motivation is inherently a historical one. The Confederate general statues that many want removed are, after all, mostly depictions of men on horseback or wielding swords, which in and of themselves are neither white supremacist nor degrading or disrespectful to African Americans. One needs the historical context of the Confederacy in order to see them in these bad lights. But no history at all is necessary for motivations to remove the Emancipation Memorial. One path of reconciliation might be to claim that Lincoln was not a racial egalitarian, which he wasn't,[18] and that this particular statue depicts his real, condescending attitude toward freed slaves and should be removed for that reason, although he did issue the Emancipation Proclamation.

The general motivation for removal is that public monuments that depict African Americans in demeaning ways—whether because of the historical context they evoke, or how they look, or because of something else about their presentation or context—ought to be removed from public view. Concerning the purported aim of those who want to remove certain statues and monuments from public view, let's consider a hypothetical: Suppose nothing else changed except that the statues under contention were removed. Would this correct past racial oppression or contemporary racism? It is difficult for anyone to believe it would. The absence of the statues in a society that many people of color consider racist and oppressive against them would make it seem on the surface of public spaces as though slave owners and White Supremacists never were honored, and as though it were not the case that public symbols of their honor are the price that people of color have had to pay for the formal liberatory gains of the civil rights movements. The statue-removing efforts and counter-insistence to keep them in place are a worthwhile rhetorical exercise, an occasion to discuss history in a culture that has little interest in its history, apart from this issue. This is why moving the contentious statues to museums would not accomplish anything either. Americans have to make special efforts to go to museums and learn about the historical artifacts displayed within them.

But having contentious statues on display, under threat of removal, does capture the popular interest and imagination. Thus, the period of time in which the statues are on display, and their acceptance or controversy, is also part of history, which records important facets of public attitudes at different times. This account of some of the statue removal motivation and its historical blind spots, together with how the *New York Times* dealt with Tom Cotton's op-ed, highlights a recent trend that has been called *canceling*.

CANCEL CULTURE

The practice of "ghosting" may have come first, followed by shunning and shaming. Cancel culture is a trend on Twitter, Facebook, and other social media platforms, which has been described as "boycotting" an individual or organization for identified misbehavior or speech that is deemed oppressive or offensive in the present time. However, the range of miscreant behavior or speech can extend decades into the past, over the lifetime of an offending person, so anachronism does not put a brake on cancellation. As of this writing, cancellation is the most current aversive strategy when confronted with obnoxious expressive acts or people. But like ghosting as a practice in personal relationships, it is based on beliefs that growth or change in interactions are not possible.[19] Canceling is an effort to exile or blot someone or something out of shared discourse. Current cultural rhetoric quickly becomes "meta," so the subject is not whether X or Y should be canceled; instead, it is whether canceling in current contexts is valid, something that good, progressive people should be willing to do. On July 7, 2020, *Harper's* magazine published the following letter online, with a list of those who had signed it.

A Letter on Justice and Open Debate
The below letter will be appearing in the Letters section of the magazine's October issue. We welcome responses at letters@harpers.org.

Our cultural institutions are facing a moment of trial. Powerful protests for racial and social justice are leading to overdue demands for police reform, along with wider calls for greater equality and inclusion across our society, not least in higher education, journalism, philanthropy, and the arts. But this needed reckoning has also intensified a new set of moral attitudes and political commitments that tend to weaken our norms of open debate and toleration of differences in favor of ideological conformity. As we applaud the first development, we also raise our voices against the second. The forces of illiberalism are gaining strength throughout the world and have a powerful ally in Donald Trump, who represents a real threat to democracy. But resistance must not be allowed to harden into its own brand of dogma or coercion—which right-wing demagogues are already exploiting. The democratic inclusion we want can be achieved only if we speak out against the intolerant climate that has set in on all sides.

The free exchange of information and ideas, the lifeblood of a liberal society, is daily becoming more constricted. While we have come to expect this on the radical right, censoriousness is also spreading more widely in our culture: an intolerance of opposing views, a vogue for public shaming and ostracism, and the tendency to dissolve complex policy issues in a blinding moral certainty. We uphold the value of robust and even caustic counter-speech from all quarters. But it is now all too common to hear calls for swift and severe retribution in response to perceived transgressions of speech and thought. More troubling still, institutional leaders, in a spirit of panicked damage control, are delivering hasty and disproportionate punishments instead of considered reforms. Editors are fired for running controversial pieces; books are withdrawn for alleged inauthenticity; journalists are barred from writing on certain topics; professors are investigated for quoting works of literature in class; a researcher is fired for circulating a peer-reviewed academic study; and the heads of organizations are ousted for what are sometimes just clumsy mistakes. Whatever the arguments around each particular incident, the result has been to steadily narrow the boundaries of what can be said without the threat of reprisal. We are already paying the price in greater risk aversion among writers, artists, and journalists who fear for their livelihoods if they depart from the consensus, or even lack sufficient zeal in agreement.

This stifling atmosphere will ultimately harm the most vital causes of our time. The restriction of debate, whether by a repressive government or an intolerant society, invariably hurts those who lack power and makes everyone less capable of democratic participation. The way to defeat bad ideas is by exposure, argument, and persuasion, not by trying to silence or wish them away. We refuse any false choice between justice and freedom, which cannot exist without each other. As writers we need a culture that leaves us room for experimentation, risk taking, and even mistakes. We need to preserve the possibility of good-faith disagreement without dire professional consequences. If we won't defend the very thing on which our work depends, we shouldn't expect the public or the state to defend it for us.

Signed by: Elliot Ackerman; Saladin Ambar, Rutgers University; Martin Amis; Anne Applebaum; Marie Arana, author; Margaret Atwood; John Banville; Mia Bay, historian; Louis Begley, writer; Roger Berkowitz, Bard College; Paul Berman, writer; Sheri Berman, Barnard College; Reginald Dwayne Betts, poet; Neil Blair, agent; David W. Blight, Yale University; Jennifer Finney Boylan, author; David Bromwich; David Brooks, columnist; Ian Buruma, Bard College; Lea Carpenter; Noam Chomsky, MIT (emeritus); Nicholas A. Christakis, Yale University; Roger Cohen, writer; Ambassador Frances D. Cook, ret.; Drucilla Cornell, Founder, uBuntu Project; Kamel Daoud; Meghan Daum, writer; Gerald Early, Washington University–St. Louis; Jeffrey Eugenides, writer; Dexter Filkins; Federico Finchelstein, The New School; Caitlin Flanagan; Richard T. Ford, Stanford Law School; Kmele Foster; David Frum, journalist; Francis Fukuyama, Stanford University; Atul Gawande, Harvard University; Todd Gitlin, Columbia University; Kim Ghattas; Malcolm Gladwell; Michelle Goldberg, columnist; Rebecca Goldstein, writer; Anthony Grafton, Princeton University; David Greenberg, Rutgers University; Linda Greenhouse; Rinne B. Groff, playwright; Sarah Haider, activist; Jonathan Haidt, NYU-Stern; Roya Hakakian, writer; Shadi Hamid, Brookings Institution; Jeet Heer, The Nation; Katie Herzog, podcast host; Susannah Heschel, Dartmouth College; Adam Hochschild, author; Arlie Russell Hochschild, author; Eva Hoffman, writer; Coleman Hughes, writer/Manhattan Institute; Hussein Ibish, Arab Gulf States Institute; Michael Ignatieff; Zaid Jilani, journalist; Bill T. Jones, New York Live Arts;Wendy Kaminer, writer; Matthew Karp, Princeton University; Garry Kasparov, Renew; Democracy Initiative; Daniel Kehlmann, writer; Randall Kennedy; Khaled Khalifa, writer; Parag Khanna, author; Laura Kipnis, Northwestern University; Frances Kissling, Center for Health, Ethics, Social Policy; Enrique Krauze, historian; Anthony Kronman, Yale University; Joy Ladin, Yeshiva University; Nicholas Lemann, Columbia University; Mark Lilla, Columbia University; Susie Linfield, New York University; Damon Linker, writer; Dahlia Lithwick, Slate; Steven Lukes, New York University; John R. MacArthur, publisher, writer; Susan Madrak, writer; Phoebe Maltz Bovy, writer; Greil Marcus; Wynton Marsalis, Jazz at Lincoln Center; Kati Marton, author; Debra Mashek, scholar; Deirdre McCloskey, University of Illinois at Chicago; John McWhorter, Columbia University; Uday Mehta, City University of New York; Andrew Moravcsik, Princeton University; Yascha Mounk, Persuasion; Samuel Moyn, Yale University; Meera Nanda, writer and teacher; Cary Nelson, University of Illinois at Urbana–Champaign; Olivia Nuzzi, New York Magazine; Mark Oppenheimer, Yale University; Dael Orlandersmith, writer/performer; George Packer; Nell Irvin Painter, Princeton University (emerita); Greg Pardlo, Rutgers University–Camden; Orlando Patterson, Harvard University; Steven Pinker, Harvard University; Letty Cottin Pogrebin; Katha Pollitt, writer; Claire Bond Potter, The New School; Taufiq Rahim; Zia Haider Rahman, writer; Jennifer Ratner-Rosenhagen, University of Wisconsin; Jonathan Rauch, Brookings Institution/The Atlantic; Neil

Roberts, political theorist; Melvin Rogers, Brown University; Kat Rosenfield, writer; Loretta J. Ross, Smith College; J. K. Rowling; Salman Rushdie, New York University; Karim Sadjadpour, Carnegie Endowment; Daryl Michael Scott, Howard University; Diana Senechal, teacher and writer; Jennifer Senior, columnist; Judith Shulevitz, writer; Jesse Singal, journalist; Anne-Marie Slaughter; Andrew Solomon, writer; Deborah Solomon, critic and biographer; Allison Stanger, Middlebury College; Paul Starr, American Prospect/Princeton University; Wendell Steavenson, writer; Gloria Steinem, writer and activist; Nadine Strossen, New York Law School; Ronald S. Sullivan Jr., Harvard Law School; Kian Tajbakhsh, Columbia University; Zephyr Teachout, Fordham University; Cynthia Tucker, University of South Alabama; Adaner Usmani, Harvard University; Chloe Valdary; Helen Vendler, Harvard University; Judy B. Walzer; Michael Walzer; Eric K. Washington, historian; Caroline Weber, historian; Randi Weingarten, American Federation of Teachers; Bari Weiss; Sean Wilentz, Princeton University; Garry Wills; Thomas Chatterton Williams, writer; Robert F. Worth, journalist and author; Molly Worthen, University of North Carolina at Chapel Hill; Matthew Yglesias; Emily Yoffe, journalist; Cathy Young, journalist; Fareed Zakaria. *Institutions are listed for identification purposes only.* [20]

The *Harper's* letter is fairly bland. It invokes principles of free expression and advises that progressives should not imitate the strategies of censorship and denial against which they are struggling. However, as noted, public discourse has become sophisticated, now including what it should include in discussions about itself and who is a reliable discussant. And so the foregoing *Harper's* letter, insofar as it was an attack on or criticism of cancel culture, was met with an effort to cancel it. Thus, in the *Los Angeles Times*, two days later, from Mary McNamara, culture columnist and critic: "'Cancel culture' is not the problem. The *Harper's* letter is." McNamara characterizes the letter as "yet another term used as a blanket criticism of people, often young but not always, deploying new forms of communication (in this case, social media) to call out those they believe are espousing or enabling racism, sexism, homophobia, transphobia, sexual harassment and capitalistic exploitation. (Or, less grandly, to promote inter-influencer feuds.)"

McNamara also taunted the *Harper's* letter signers for seeking to protect a man who had a screaming meltdown in Costco because he didn't want to wear a mask, as well as Tom Cotton and the *New York*

Times op-ed editor who was fired for running his piece. She also mentions earlier criticism of *Harper's* letter signer J. K. Rowling's apparent implication that trans women are not really women. McNamara's strongest claim in terms of left politics is that "the supposed cancelers have little or no institutional power," so that "all they have is the influence of the collective."[21]

McNamara's criticism of the *Harper's* letter is a criticism of those who advocate free speech for intolerant and reactionary opponents, even though the advocates are on the morally right side and their beliefs are based on facts. This is Mill's argument all over again, made concrete in our own time. The argument against the *New York Times* failing to provide a forum where people can disagree with morally correct and factually accurate claims and aims has already been mentioned in the previous section. If someone who doesn't want to wear a mask in a pandemic is allowed to express themselves, why is that not an opportunity to re-explain the issue and try to understand their resistance? Because J. K. Rowling insisted that "sex is real," does this mean that she has nothing to say about free speech?[22]

The claim that those with little institutional power are justified in silencing disagreement within their own ranks raises interesting issues about political rhetoric that go beyond social media. Indeed, the *Harper's* letter signers are correct in claiming that jobs have been lost and employers pressured by the overhanging fear of canceling as it verges into boycotting. (McNamara approves of the latter, citing United Farm Workers.) Thus, canceling acquires the urgency of activism for a just cause. But what about all of the intervening discussion and airing of views that helps people form their final opinions and resolve to act for a just cause? It is in that rhetorical space where we might want to take care that we don't hold our righteous opinions as mere prejudices. And the best way of doing that is to have the patience to participate in, or listen to, or read views and arguments (if they have any) counter to those opinions.

From a morally good and progressive social and political perspective, much is oppressive in the actions and speech of individuals, organizations, and businesses. We—that is, "we enlightened or 'woke' ones"—know that such reports, public displays, and character flaws are reprehensible and dangerous for young minds and sensibilities. The problem is what to do about them. The removal of bad ideas by news publishers, the removal of Confederate statues in public spaces, and cancellations in social media share a reaction of banishing, obscuring, or refusing to mention or interact with that which is offensive. There are obvious reasons for not practicing this kind of reaction. It is like closing one's eyes so as not to see something unpleasant, knowing full well that the unpleasantness remains, out of sight, but also believing that not looking is a way to deal with what one does not want to see. If the sole raison d'être of the object one refuses to see is that one see it, then not looking can be an effective way to deal with it. But that is seldom the case, and usually what we don't want to see has come into existence for reasons independent of our reactions.

Of course, anyone is within their rights to choose not to attend to what offends them, but it is mistaken to believe that such choice obliterates the offending object. If a rhetorical space is cleared (that is, sanitized of what is offensive), then that detritus does cease to exist in that space. If tolerated to remain in the rhetorical space, it is possible that there could be change, growth, or even conversion. But once banished from one's own rhetorical space, the offensive person or idea only ceases to exist in one's own rhetorical space and may take up life in another rhetorical space, where one does not know what goes on. To quote from the *Harper's* letter reprinted above, *"The way to defeat bad ideas is by exposure, argument, and persuasion, not by trying to silence or wish them away."*

As we saw in chapter 1, the SARS-CoV-2 virus can be destroyed by sanitization, but sanitization in one place is not contagious in the way that the virus is contagious. The intact iterations of the virus remain in existence where they have not been sanitized away. Some of the heightened removals, banishments, and cancellations in this time of COVID-19 may be symbolic reactions of what we would collectively like to happen to SARS-CoV-2, a displaced, symbolic enactment of control over the virus that we do not actually have but wish we did have.

The latter is reminiscent of Sigmund Freud's grandson, Ernst, who played the game of Fort-Da (Here! There!). At eighteen months, Ernst would deliberately hide and then find small objects. His behavior and Freud's interpretation have been much discussed in psychoanalytic literature. Was Ernst taking revenge on his parents for leaving him and then returning? Was he symbolically taking control of emotionally painful issues of loss or abandonment? Was he learning the use of symbols and playing with them?[23] Of course, Ernst had every reason to rely on the sameness or constancy of the objects he first banished or hid and then rediscovered. He had no reason to fear that they would reappear to him as larger, or more dangerous, or greater in number. But in a volatile situation such as the present, we do not have that constancy. Hence, the second epigraph to this chapter from the movie *The Godfather: Part II*—"Keep your friends close, but your enemies closer."

9

CONSPIRACY

"A video touting an unfounded conspiracy theory that Bill Gates is behind the coronavirus outbreak has gone viral on Instagram with the help of the accounts of celebrities such as Cedric the Entertainer, D. L. Hughley and Derrick Lewis, a mixed martial artist."
—Brandy Zadrozny, NBC News contributor[1]

"Apparently I have the Wuhan [*sic*] virus . . . and I don't know about everybody, but when I have a mask on I'm moving it to make it comfortable, and I can't help but wonder if that put some germs in the mask. Keep your hands off your mask? Anyway, who knows?"
—Louie Gohmert (US House of Representatives, R-Texas)[2]

"It is not, perhaps, amiss to relieve or enliven a busy scene sometimes with such digressions, whether to the purpose or no."
—John Locke, *Essay Concerning Human Understanding*, 1689[3]

The new importance of news in a default role of entertainment during quarantines can represent a blurring of imagination and reality-based thought, or a substitution of fiction for nonfiction. The enhanced role of rhetoric, as discussed in earlier chapters, also blurs the boundary between reality and fabrication. US literature includes well-entrenched genres of spy and political thrillers, as well as dystopian science fiction. During COVID-19, the distinction between scenarios from the realm of imagination and descriptions of reality has become blurred in conspiracy theories. For COVID-19, as for other disasters or shocking disruptive events, conspiracy theories posit secret agreements among powerful people as their ultimate causes. The evidence for such conspiracies usually comes from the disaster itself, cast as an effect of a deliberate plan, conceived by people or organizations with sufficient power to implement it. Their motives are posited as political power, insatiable desire for greater wealth, or malevolence against humanity or some specific group therein.

Some conspiracy theories pertaining to COVID-19 derive from more total worldviews that were in circulation before the pandemic. It is rare for such conspiracy theories to provide evidence of an actual meeting or series of meetings or even communication about the subject among conspirators. It may be enough if they have had opportunities to meet in person through their normal business activity; barring that, there is always electronic communication. Elite invitation-only groups have become obvious and usual suspects. One example has been the Bilderberg group, named after a 1954 meeting at the Hotel de Bilderberg in Oosterbeek, Netherlands. By the 1960s, many took it for granted that its members were involved in plotting "The New World Order."[4]

COVID-19 conspiracies have ranged from Marxist-type "follow the money" conjectures about who stands to benefit from the pandemic, such as those who are already billionaires (primarily Bill Gates), to bizarre scenarios that seem to educated people to have been formulated purely for distraction, amusement, or cheap thrills. In addition to well-developed conspiracy theories, COVID-19 has generated much misinformation, including moneymaking schemes in the online marketplace. The first section of this chapter introduces some widespread misinformation and bogus products sold and includes discussion of dismissal, which is not yet full-blown denial. Next comes a consideration of well-developed conspiracy theories that circulated during the first six months of the pandemic. Finally, there is discussion of the epistemology involved in taking conspiracy theories seriously and the profound ignorance of science and lack of critical thinking skills thereby implied. The thin line between belief in conspiracy and suspicion during a pandemic that has been politicized is considered. Along the way, there is an ongoing attempt not to overstate arguments against misinformation and conspiracy theories, because those who are "right" are not without our own biases.

MISINFORMATION ABOUT COVID-19

Not all forms of misinformation are conspiracy theories, but most forms have the effect of distraction from actually solving practical problems. Some misinformation is profitable for its purveyors. Those who accept factual misinformation about COVID-19 believe that the disease is real and threatening but diverge from official science-based accounts of how best to address it. At the beginning of the COVID-19 pandemic, some African Americans circulated a rumor that they were immune to the SARS-CoV-2 virus, because it was an exclusively white disease or an old person's disease. At that time, the patients who received publicity were mostly white and old, and, statistically, there is a higher proportion of young people in the black community.[5] There is nothing about SARS-CoV-2 or about African Americans that would confirm their immunity. In fact, due to working conditions and preexisting medical conditions resulting from preexisting neglect of their health by the medical and public health communities, African Americans may be suffering more than any other racial or ethnic group, except, perhaps, Latinx Americans (see chapter 4).

False cures for COVID-19 are a combination of individual gullibility and distrust of science, as well as opportunistic greed. By early August 2020, the FDA provided a list of ninety-five products with a statement of its intent to interrupt their sale:

> The FDA is exercising its authority to protect consumers from firms selling unapproved products and making false or misleading claims, including, by pursuing warning letters, seizures, injunctions or criminal prosecutions against products and firms or individuals that violate the law.[6]

Wikipedia is probably more up to date with its list of more than 147 sources. COVID-19 commerce and misinformation on social media have proliferated, amounting to a whack-a-mole type problem. Products advertised have included disinfectants with less than the 70 percent alcohol required to remove the virus; bogus advice about gargling, nasal rinsing, and inhaling, sometimes with toxic ingredients; inadequate protective equipment; bogus health exercises and dietary practices; magical practices; phony diagnostic kits; and expensive but ineffective light and electronic devices.[7]

In June 2020, the US Environmental Protection Agency issued stop-sale orders to Amazon.com and eBay about false claims for products from third parties, with a threat of fines over $20,000 per sale.[8] It remains to be reported whether this approach will be an effective deterrent and how many billions of dollars this industry will gross.

There are no proven substances to prevent COVID-19 contagion, except for the mechanical avoidance measures of social distancing, mask wearing, and hand and surface washing. The medical care for those requiring hospitalization is largely supportive, although Remdesivir and steroid treatments, as well as antibiotic therapies for secondary infections, are increasing in use as supplies are manufactured and become available. Also in use are convalescent plasma or antibodies from recovering COVID-19 patients; pronation, or positioning patients on their fronts to increase lung capacity; and supplemental oxygen. Ventilators and extracorporeal membrane oxygenation (ECMO), which oxygenates blood outside of the body, are further therapies for serious and critical cases.[9]

If misinformation comes from an otherwise respected expert, it requires correction by other experts. In April 2020, it was widely reported that Luc Montagnier, a Nobel Prize winner for his co-discovery of the AIDS virus, was claiming that SARS-CoV-2 was a genetically engineered virus that had escaped from the Wuhan laboratory. Montagnier referred to analyses showing that SARS-CoV-2 had genetic sequences from the AIDS virus and SARS-CoV-1. He concluded that SARS-CoV-2 was the result of failed attempts to make an AIDS vaccine. However, studies of the SARS-CoV-2 virus have led critics of Montagnier's thesis to point out that this virus has a distinct spike enabling it to latch onto human immune-regulating cells, which is likely the result of a natural change in the evolution of the virus. The spike on the SARS-CoV-2 virus is different from the spike on the SARS-CoV-1 virus, and that would have enabled more straightforward cellular binding in laboratory manipulation, thereby making it unnecessary to genetically engineer SARS-CoV-2. Moreover, the genetic sequence in common with the AIDS virus is a common sequence, believed to have evolved ten thousand years ago.[10]

Finally, some Americans persist in attitudes of big misinformation about COVID-19. They do not accept the reality of COVID-19 and may or may not subscribe to conspiracy theories. Because they do not accept that COVID-19 is real, they may believe that reports about it are purely political, from sources they oppose (e.g., the Democratic Party). They may believe that COVID-19 is no worse than a flu, or, based on their own experience, that it simply does not exist. This is an attitude of dismissal, rather than denial, and it can be summed up something like this:

> Some people believe there is a disease called COVID-19 but no one I know has caught it and reports of illness and death from it have been contested. If there is such a disease, it's more like a flu. There-fore, I'm not worried about catching it and intend to go on with my life.

On April 10, 2020, the *New York Times* reported interviews with attendees at a motorcycle rally in Sturgis, South Dakota, which was projected to draw 250,000. Here is a sampling of comments from differ-ent attendees regarding their presence at what experts feared would be a "super-spreader event" in the ongoing pandemic:

> I come to meet up with old friends, people I haven't seen in forever and a lot of folks I grew up with. . . . But I don't know one person in a six-state radius who has had COVID. I think it is all just political.

> We got married here three years ago, so we come out here every year for our anniversary. Now we have a reason to come here every year.

> We have no concerns—if we are going to get sick, then we'll get sick.

> I'm not convinced it's real. I think it's nothing more than the flu. If I die from the virus, it was just meant to be.

> I come out every year. This is my first year staying on the Island. I was invited in by my cousin. The people here, we have become extended family.

> You've got to be smart. I've got masks. When I walk around or ride around, I wear a mask. [11]

While not representative, in a scientific sense, of all 250,000 attend-ees, these comments are interesting for the way they disclose individual motivations and attitudes. They indicate that meeting friends and family were some of the reasons for attending, and they also reveal a dismissal of the reality of COVID-19. If dismissal were not a pervasive attitude, more masks would have been in evidence, so they could be said to be blocking or denying the pandemic by their actions. Both their words and their actions were blithe. That is, attendees did not go to Sturgis despite COVID-19, although motivated by social loyalties, but with an attitude that COVID-19 is not a real disaster.

Finally, there have also been factual scientific reports that, taken together, are ambiguous. For instance, early in the COVID-19 pandemic, smoking was listed as a preexisting condition that could increase the destructive effects of the disease. But soon after, studies showed a lower than usual number of smokers in China who required treatment for COVID-19, given their percentage in the population. Many scientists continued to advise against both smoking and vaping during the pandemic. But others reported that nicotine has the ability to block the virus from latching onto immune reaction regulation cells, which would block contagion or serious illness, and they speculated that nicotine could be included in treatment options.[12] Still, the American Cancer Society has not revised its advisory from April 2020, which is consistent with established warnings about smoking:

> Currently, the US Centers for Disease Control and Prevention (CDC) states, "Being a current or former cigarette smoker may increase your risk of severe illness from COVID-19." And according to the WHO, "Smoking impairs lung function, making it harder for the body to fight off coronaviruses and other respiratory diseases. Available research suggests that smokers are at higher risk of developing severe COVID-19 outcomes and death."[13]

POPULAR CONSPIRACY THEORIES

Conspiracy theories are narratives that may be part of wider worldviews, and their authors often have wider experience before focusing on COVID-19. We will focus on 5G and "Plandemic" in this sense.

5G at 60 GHz

The cell-phone technology of 5G as a cause of COVID-19 was discussed in an April 2020 interview with British conspiracy theorist David Vaughan Icke. According to Icke, 5G poisons the cells in a human body and the cells then release *exosomes*. When the real-time polymerase chain reaction (RT-PCR) test is used on an individual, they then test positive for COVID-19, purely as a result of the 5G-induced exosomes. Furthermore, 5G at 60 gigahertz (GHz) can actually stop the human body from absorbing oxygen into the blood, which interferes with lung functioning. And that is the impairment of lung functioning, which scientists have attributed to the action of SARS-CoV-2 in the human respiratory system.

Icke's account is meant to explain the phenomenon of COVID-19, but it is part of his more comprehensive worldview. He has previously claimed that the world is run by an elite system called the *Illuminati*, who include the British government and royal family and a large number of celebrities and journalists. The Illuminati are descended from, or possessed by, alien lizard-type people who can shape-shift as they drink blood and sacrifice children. Icke's COVID-19 speculations were removed by Facebook and YouTube as misinformation likely to damage public health.[14]

In reality, GHz is a measure of electromagnetic frequency, and exposure to 60 GHz is similar to sunlight exposure, but at 1/10,000 of the energy.[15] A 2019 review of experimental studies concluded that 5G–60 GHz is within a frequency range that does not cause thermal damage to living things.[16] In rumors circulating on social media in Nigeria, Tanzania, Bolivia, Egypt, and the United Kingdom, it was claimed that 5G mobile phone masts cause COVID-19. The International Fact-Checking Network (IFCN) has reported its attempts to debunk this theory in at least fourteen countries that include Greece, Kazakhstan, the Philippines, and Mexico.

In Argentina, a YouTube video promoting the conspiracy theory had 1.3 million views; in Pakistan, a video had 650,000 views. This speculation, some of it circulated by religious and political leaders, as well as celebrities, has not only caused anxiety but also motivated attempts to destroy cell masts—even in places where there has been no 5G technology. Bill Gates has been portrayed as a major villain in this conspiracy for planning to have microchips implanted into human beings when they are vaccinated against the virus; the microchips are supposed to be linked to individuals' social media profiles in order to control them. Conspiracy promoters in different locales insert their own cultural interpretations. For example, in Arabic versions, the implants were called "Antichrist chips."[17]

Still, not all areas of the world have fact checkers or credible voices against the 5G conspiracy theory. John Oliver inimitably debunked the 5G theory on July 19, 2020, by attacking apparent evidence for it. The evidence is that COVID-19 outbreaks have been most intense in areas with 5G service. Indeed, the maps of both 5G geographical usage and COVID-19 cases are remarkably similar. Oliver pointed out that such places are also densely populated, which causes rapid contagion. The YouTube version of Oliver's show, "Conspiracy Theories," had over five million views in its first five days. Whether these were from people eager for Oliver's debunking information, or searching for more information about the 5G conspiracy, is an open question.[18]

5G and Hydroxychloroquine

Like SARS-CoV-2, conspiracy theories do not simply go away. Attacking one conspiracy theory may leave intact roots entangled with the roots of other conspiracy theories. In April 2020, 5G conspiracists had already connected 5G damage with hydroxychloroquine, the drug discredited as a cure for COVID-19.[19] Hydroxychloroquine had initially been touted by President Trump as a powerful "game changer," a view endorsed by President Bolsonaro of Brazil, who reported taking the drug before and during his own COVID-19 illness. Sixty-three million doses of hydroxychloroquine were added to the Strategic National Stockpile, at taxpayer expense.[20] Despite its combined failure to cure COVID-19, harmful side effects in some patients, and the Food and Drug Administration's (FDA) withdrawal of its authorization for emergency use,[21] Trump resurrected his promotion of hydroxychloroquine in an approving reference to a quite spectacular conspiracy theorist, Dr. Stella Immanuel.

Dr. Immanuel, who practices at Rehoboth Medical Center, a clinic in Houston, has claimed not only that hydroxychloroquine cures COVID-19 but also that its use was being suppressed by "Big Pharma" and Bill Gates, pending an eventual vaccine that would contain a substance causing its recipients to forego their religion. Immanuel has also propounded theories that many women's gynecological problems are the result of sexual assault by "astral spirit men." She is the leader of a group called "America's Frontline Doctors" who participated in an event organized by Tea Party Patriots Action, a "dark money group" that has helped fund a pro-Trump political action committee. This event, in which members of the group posed in white coats, was video-recorded, and President Trump retweeted that video.[22] (It is not often noted that even if Immanuel were correct about the vaccine conspiracy, vaccines would confer immunity, whereas hydroxychloroquine is supposed to be an antiviral treatment, and it did not confer immunity on Bolsonaro.)

After pushback on both the efficacy of hydroxychloroquine and Dr. Immanuel's credibility, Trump defended his retweet of the video: "I think they're very respected doctors. There was a woman who was spectacular in her statements about it."[23] Pop icon Madonna also lent her voice to this chorus, hailing Immanuel as her "hero" in a tweet that Instagram took down for its misinformation:

> The Truth will set us all Free! But some people don't want to hear the truth. Especially the people in power who stand to make money from this long drawn out search for a vaccine.[24]

Plandemic

The Plandemic conspiracy theory is an intersection of preexisting anti-vaxxer beliefs with a theory about the origin of SARS-CoV-2. The anti-vaxxer community has developed influence through social media in recent decades, based on anecdotal evidence that vaccines cause autism and chronic fatigue syndrome. Many anti-vaxxers also believe that vaccines are made available to the public as part of a government plot to increase surveillance and control, in addition to enriching big pharmaceutical companies. As a result of anti-vaxxer influence, there is concern in the medical community that should there be a safe and effective vaccine conferring immunity against SARS-CoV-2, many will refuse to take it. This will delay herd immunity, which will stop the disease in the United States after a critical percentage of the population (between 60 and 90 percent) is immune,[25] although others may delay getting vaccinated until an available vaccine has proved safe as well as effective.

The twenty-six-minute video *Plandemic*, an interview with Judy Mikovits, PhD (a virologist who became famous on alt-right media during the early spring of 2020), was soon taken down from YouTube and became difficult to access.[26] Mikovits had worked on AIDS research with Dr. Anthony Fauci several decades ago. Mikovits's claims made in the video are partly developed in an earlier book (number-one seller on Amazon during attention to the video). Mikovits co-wrote *Plague: One Scientist's Intrepid Search for the Truth about Human Retroviruses and Chronic Fatigue Syndrome (ME/CFS), Autism, and Other Diseases* with Kent Heckenlively, an anti-vaxxer authority. The central claim of this book is that chronic fatigue syndrome, autism, and other new diseases were caused by viruses in vaccines. A conspiracy was posited that treatment for these diseases, as well as for HIV, was delayed in the 1980s and 1990s until unscrupulous doctors and drug companies could get patents for those treatments. Mikovits may also have begun the rumor that COVID-19 death rates were inflated to increase the need for said patented vaccine.[27]

Claims from Mikovits's interview were answered in detail in the *New York Times* and other media, as well as by Mikhail Varshavski, DO (aka "Dr. Mike"), a doctor of osteopathy in family practice in New York City.[28] (Mikovits also made claims about her own unjust arrest and damage to her career due to speaking out against Dr. Fauci, but these are not relevant to COVID-19.) It is worthwhile to consider Mikovits's main claims about COVID-19 together with Dr. Mike's rebuttals, because his responses are accessible to nonscientists, and he regularly has as many viewers as the *Plandemic* video first received.[29]

Dr. Mike pointed out that Dr. Mikovits's claim that Bill Gates and Anthony Fauci conspired to allow COVID-19 to spread and suppressed the development of a vaccine until they could secure patents for it is self-contradictory. Widespread contagion would result in herd immunity. Dr. Mike points out that there is no evidence of falsified death certificates and that medical causes of death are often multiple, as a matter of course. (Also, epidemiologists have reported that COVID-19 deaths may be higher than official figures, which often do not include deaths in nursing homes or home deaths.)[30] Mikovits asserted that doctors are paid $13,000 for each COVID-19 patient and $39,000 for ventilator treatment, which she deemed unjust enrichment. Dr. Mike pointed out that hospitals are paid based on average costs that are set by Medicare/Medicaid cost-saving practices over a range of diseases. Mikovits asserted the Wuhan lab–origin theory, and Dr. Mike pointed out that this has been disputed by further scientific investigation. Mikovits asserted that elderly people in Italy had received flu shots for multiple flu strains that had been cultivated in dog saliva, which has many coronaviruses and thereby gave people SARS-CoV-2. Dr. Mike pointed out that there is no evidence that patients got COVID-19 from vaccines cultured in dog saliva, where coronaviruses present are benign.

Mikovits also asserted that the human immune system is damaged by lockdown measures that cause illnesses to shoot up when people finally go outside. She also said that wearing a mask causes people to "activate their own coronavirus." Dr. Mike pointed out that immunity doesn't work that way. The immune systems of people in hygienic bubbles for long periods of time are likely to overreact when exposed to pathogens, not underreact. There is no evidence that masks "activate" a person's own virus, or even a plausible explanation of what that could mean. (Dr. Mike could have added that there is no evidence that SARS-CoV-2 can be dormant within the human body, so that it could be "activated.")

Mikovits claimed that only patented medications are used in hospitals, so that drug companies can make money; this arrangement drives out older remedies that might work just as well, but more cheaply. Dr. Mike pointed out that it cost a lot of money for the research and trials necessary to develop new drugs. However, Bill Gates and several large drug companies have pledged to donate any vaccines they discover. Moreover, modern medicine based on patented drugs works better than older remedies, even if they are cheaper. (However, antacid medication was said to work as a treatment for COVID-19 when it was used by poor people in Wuhan, who could not afford more expensive treatments.[31])[32]

Sinclair Broadcast Group is a media company that owns or operates 294 television stations across the United States, with 89 markets that range in size from Washington, DC, to small towns in Iowa and Missouri. Sinclair's news is often blended with editorial comments in line with what President Trump claims about COVID-19. Sinclair Broadcasting stations were poised to run an interview with Dr. Mikovits in late July

2020, but they pulled it due to strong objections against furthering misinformation about COVID-19, which could damage public health.[33]

Virologists have sought to determine the origin of the COVID-19 pandemic by sequencing its genome and those of similar viruses. A consensus has been reached that bats are the origin of the virus SARS-CoV-2, because there is a similarity between the SARS-CoV-2 virus and bat viruses, although there had been US State Department concern about the high-containment laboratory, the Wuhan Institute for Virology. Past accidental exposures of the influenza virus and SARS-CoV (the SARS virus) led to concern that SARS-CoV-2 may have escaped from the Wuhan laboratory. However, natural emergence from bat populations was assessed to be more likely in the absence of evidence for laboratory escape.

This hypothesis also received more support than the hypothesis of wildlife market origins. Although there were positive COVID-19 cases in the environment of the Wuhan "wet market," none of the animal samples from the Wuhan wet market tested positive for SARS-CoV-2. This result put to rest the earlier wet market account of the disease origin. Evidence of viral circulation in November 2019, before evidence of the virus in the environment of the Wuhan wet market, further complicated the wet market account.[34]

THE EPISTEMOLOGY OF CONSPIRACY THEORIES

In philosophy, epistemology is an account of the grounds for, and nature of, knowledge. Epistemology begins with the assumption that there is knowledge or beliefs that are true. Speaking of the epistemology of belief in conspiracy theories requires reverse engineering the thought processes and motivations that could result in their construction and acceptance. But insofar as conspiracy theories of the nature that have just been displayed are not knowledge, they have no "epistemology," but perhaps psychology instead. The emptiness of knowledge in the "conspirasphere" would be the first psycho-epistemological problem.

People who believe in conspiracy theories do not begin with ideas of what it takes to know something and what kinds of assertions can count as knowledge. In an anti-intellectual and anti-expert culture, there may not be much value placed on knowledge, under that name. But presumably, people who believe in conspiracy theories think that some things are true while others are not. They grasp the idea that some news accounts may not be true—hence their participation in the Republican or conservative appropriation of the label "fake news," which was originally used by Democrats and progressives to dismiss false news reports circulated on social media. But if conspiracy believers seek what is true, they do not consistently follow a method of either critical or logical thinking or adherence to known facts. If a method for arriving at the truth is not deemed necessary, or even imagined to exist, then the content of an account or description alone becomes sufficient for believing it. It may be enough for conspiracy subscribers if a story or narrative appeals to them or is consistent with their other beliefs or what their friends and relatives believe.

Part of the conspiracist rejection of knowledge is undoubtedly connected to a mistrust of scientific and other expert opinion. Experts are those who know more about a specific subject than others who have not studied it as long or to the same degree. Scientists use shared methodologies with others in their fields. Scientific findings are peer-reviewed, a process that can include duplication of experiments, consideration of alternate hypotheses and explanations, and critical assessment of conclusions. The general scientific method is supposed to yield conclusions that are probably true, to high degrees.

But because conclusions depend on data and consideration of alternative hypotheses and conclusions, they are never 100 percent certain. Science is able to keep growing because the methods and conclusions in different fields are subject to revision as new hypotheses are formed and new data become available. This unstable nature of science, which is integral to its progress, is difficult to understand by people who have not systematically studied a specialized field. In a word, conspiracy theories are themselves amateurish—they do not arise out of systematic study in a community of specialists. And the nonprofessional origins of conspiracy theories do not concern those who believe them.

Of course, science is not completely objective, because individual practitioners and whole fields work under general paradigms (for instance, the germ theory of disease). Also, the most accomplished according to their peers, as well as the most prestigious, have undue influence. Undue influence is likewise at work among groups who are trusting of science and progressive in their perspectives concerning societal issues. There are fashions, waves, and "tipping points," and "influencers" among those who would not otherwise subscribe to conspiracy theories, as well as those who might. For instance, during the summer surge in COVID-19 cases, many prominent people, including some governors, began to encourage mask wearing.[35] And in early April 2020, the belief that President Trump had mismanaged the pandemic tipped into a majority opinion in the United States.[36]

Many believe the "right things" for the wrong reason that everyone they know believes them, so independent thinking is not a sharp distinction between the psycho-epistemologies of those who trust science and those who believe in conspiracy theories. But there is an important difference between, on the one hand, believing something because its content is appealing and knowing only the content and, on the other hand, believing it because one knows (at least approximately) how the conclusion was reached.

For example, consider "Big pharma is behind the COVID-19 pandemic" and "SARS-CoV-2 has resulted in a pandemic because it is a highly contagious virus." The first statement assigns cause and blame, which are quasi-emotional assessments and reactions, whereas the second raises more questions that require factual answers (for instance, "How does contagion occur, and how can contagion be limited?"). This kind of contrast and the villainization and even demonization of the human causes of the COVID-19 pandemic suggest that, in addition to their emotional appeal, conspiracy theories appeal to those who do not have the patience to become better informed, as guided by experts. Conspiracy believers may also be guided by personal experience, without an understanding of the distinction of how such experience may or may not be generally validated. For instance, many have claimed that hydroxychloroquine has helped them or someone they know without taking into account the distinction between anecdotal experience and clinical trials.

However, conclusions from clinical trials can be reversed by subsequent clinical trials. Science is constantly self-correcting and self-revising. This problem is compounded by the fact that most who trust science do not have the time, expertise, or background information to consult scientific sources in the reputable journals in which they appear. Instead, they rely on popularized versions of such findings, so there is a double "trust" involved. Moreover, to trust the presentations of relevant scientific findings is often to rely on an *appeal to authority*, which is a basic fallacy in informal logic.[37] We should not accept something as true because a respected authority says it is true; rather, we should have our own, more direct reasons. The majority of the informed (science-trusting) public are now captive to this fallacy of appeal to authority. But it is not only, all things considered, the best epistemological condition for the public but also a fallacy to be hoped that our elected officials can be relied upon to commit.[38] This is because what we ought or ought not to do is limited by what we can or cannot do. Those of us who are not virologists or other relevant specialists cannot do our own research or even fruitfully read primary research publications. As a result, we are cognitively dependent on those who provide us with translations into layperson's language. We have no choice but to trust these "popularizers" of science. Moral epistemology thus becomes a matter of trust.

Overall, most conspiracy theories stop after substituting "real" causes of disturbing events that are different from realistically posited ones. Those who subscribe to them are loath to accept unwanted events that occur by coincidence, incompetence, accident, natural processes, or small precipitating events that build into major disasters if not addressed in the beginning, which were all causes of the SARS-CoV-2 pandemic. The result is that no matter how nefarious the fabricated "real" causes, descriptions of unwanted events can shift to amazement at how they came about. This is a form of denial, because the focus on "real" causes can thus be strangely reassuring, or at least distracting from unwanted reality: "If people with that kind of power are behind this, there is nothing I can do, so I really don't have to do anything."

There is also a focus for blame, as though blame, even justified, repairs existing destruction—as though establishing that a fire has been caused by arson is enough to put out the flames. Other conspiracy theories are simply wishful thinking. For instance, after President Trump announced that he had contracted COVID-19 and was entering Walter Reed Hospital, followers of QAnon (the "big tent conspiracy theory" that falsely promotes the existence of a shadowy cabal of Democratic pedophiles) speculated that he was sequestering himself so that an arrest of Hillary Clinton for pedophilia could be carried out. They asserted that when Trump tweeted "We will get through this together," what he meant was "to get her [Clinton]."[39]

However, not all conspiracy theories have the qualities of stopping with causes and blame. Some may be the result of a kind of paranoia that results when people who want to understand something simply do not have enough information. So they fill in gaps from their worst fears or most pessimistic views of reality. Such otherwise good faith that is psychologically distorted sometimes makes it difficult to identify a conspiracy theory as such. For example, "Has the Trump administration deliberately downplayed the severity of the COVID-19 pandemic in the United States so as to minimize its disruption to the economy in an election year?" Difficult realities do create rational fears, and even rational fears may feed on themselves.

The difficult reality of COVID-19, together with a president who has a grandiose and inflated view of his own power, led some to fear that President Trump would invoke the Secret Powers Act of 1975. In a *New York Times* opinion piece on July 23, 2020, Gary Hart, former Democratic senator from Colorado and presidential candidate, referred to a recent discovery of one hundred documents unknown to most of the US public. Hart wrote:

> We have recently come to learn of at least a hundred documents authorizing extraordinary presidential powers in the case of a national emergency, virtually dictatorial powers without congressional or judicial checks and balances. President Trump alluded to these authorities in March when he said, "I have the right to do a lot of things that people don't even know about."

Hart called for immediate congressional investigation and public hearings, adding about these powers, "We believe they may include suspension of habeas corpus, surveillance, home intrusion, arrest without a judicial warrant, collective if not mass arrests and more; some could violate constitutional protections."[40]

The alarm sounded by Hart in July 2020 was thus: "What if President Trump takes advantage of pandemic chaos such as protests and widespread illness to become the dictator many feared he would be when he was elected?" Could he do this between the election of 2020 and Inauguration Day in 2021? As of this writing (November 12, 2020), the answer seems to be that it is unlikely. But the question must be continually kept in mind based on past evidence. In mid-July 2020, Trump sent federal troops from Customs and Border Protection (CBP) to Portland, Oregon, ostensibly to protect federal property and help fight crime, but "really" to shore up his "law and order" campaign identity.[41] Trump had also promised extensions of such actions in other "Democratic cities" where local law enforcement seemed to him to be unable to contain violent protesters.[42]

What if Trump and others had deliberately impeded progress against the spread of COVID-19 so that this exact situation would be possible? What if "they" were behind the pandemic in the first place? Indeed, according to a late September 2020 Cornell University Study of thirty-eight million English-language articles written between January 1 and May 26, 2020, Trump was found to be the greatest single driver (at 37.9 percent) of what researchers called the "infodemic."[43] However, questions that proceed from worst-case projections veer into conspiracy thinking. There is a more plausible explanation for the origin of the pandemic that has an evidentiary base: it came from bats!

Similarly, there has been too much confusion within the Trump administration's reaction to COVID-19 in the United States to lend credibility to the question of whether there has been deliberate obstruction of mitigation responses—and "they" are supporting the development of vaccines, with (according to some estimates) over $5 billion of federal money by early July 2020.[44] The deployment of federal troops is unlikely to be sustainable (there are fewer than 75,000 federal agents or troops) and always subject to check from the courts. Such highly political deployment, signaled by the term "Democratic cities," is probably best understood as fodder for Trump's campaign narrative that he is "the law and order president." And again, now that Joe Biden is president-elect, there would not seem to be enough time for Trump to invoke the powers Hart discusses. However, all lawmakers and citizens should know about the content of the documents Hart refers to and understand the procedure for invoking them, if not for addressing the expiring administration, then to have as part of an arsenal of defense of democratic institutions for disruptive times in general.

Let's return now to the posit of conspiracies as causes of unwanted events. Another explanation for the appeal of this reasoning is ignorance about the ways that ongoing, normal cultural practices can result in unforeseen disasters. For example, it is well known that building over natural, water-absorbing marshes results in flooding in cities during storms and that construction that encroaches on forested areas fuels major fires.[45] Similarly, human encroachment on animal habitats results in the transmission of zoonotic viruses, which was probably the cause of COVID-19. That fossil fuel consumption and factory farming have increased the atmospheric levels of CO_2, leading to changes in climate, is a connection from normal conditions that many are unwilling or unable to grasp. The next and final chapter will turn to Climate Change, as the disaster or catastrophe for which COVID-19 may motivate preparation.

10

ETHICS OF COVID-19 AND CLIMATE CHANGE

"Obey the laws and wear the gauze. Protect your jaws from septic paws."

—Public Service Announcement, c. 1918[1]

"Blaming every single summer heat wave or extreme weather event on global warming is a stale and discredited tactic in the alarmist playbook. Objective science proves extreme weather events such as hurricanes, tornadoes, heat waves, and droughts have become less frequent and less severe as a result of the Earth's recent modest warming."

—James Taylor[2]

"Climate change is real. It is happening right now. It is the most urgent threat facing our entire species and we need to work collectively together and stop procrastinating."

—Leonardo DiCaprio[3]

COVID-19 and Climate Change are deeply connected, but also independent, because there were pandemics before COVID-19, and Climate Change could in principle occur without pandemics. As disasters that are partly due to the reactions to them, they are similar, but there are interesting contrasts in how they intersect with beliefs and societal structures. The occurrence of the COVID-19 pandemic in an era of Climate Change has compounded the puzzle of why human beings appear to be unwilling and unable to accept global existential threats.

Both the SARS-CoV-2 virus and Climate Change are extreme international dangers that share a common cause of disaster—human behavior—which human beings are collectively unwilling to change.

In both cases, there is a classic Quarantelli-type definition of disaster, in which the reaction to the disaster is part of the disaster (see chapter 1). Failing to respond to a dangerous situation that could be brought under control with adequate response magnifies the danger in both cases. Once inadequate response by others is accepted by those who are willing to respond adequately, for the willing responders, the disaster can still be externalized and addressed. But their chances of success are lowered by the absence of cooperation, if not outright obstruction. Still, the result is hypothetical, because those who would respond adequately cannot control or get rid of those who deny and refuse. Just as an inclusive attitude toward the limits of the natural world is now necessary, so is an inclusive attitude toward those who refuse to recognize those limits. Humanism and democracy, compassion and peace, require that kind of acceptance.

Thus, the issue of our contemporary disasters is twofold: What to do about the natural world, and what to do and how to think about those who refuse to accept that there are major problems and that humans have caused them. Both sides of this issue come to rest with those who recognize a problem but appear to be unwilling or unable to take action concerning it. Logic, facts, and comprehensive argument are unlikely to change the minds and behavior of those in varied phases of denial and skepticism concerning either COVID-19 or Climate Change. But on a meta-level, a depressing comparison is in order. COVID-19 is relatively simple to understand and accept compared to Climate Change. The SARS-CoV-2 virus causes the disease COVID-19, which causes death in vulnerable patients. The time between contagion and illness is about two to fourteen days. Before an effective vaccine is available, COVID-19 contagion can only be prevented by avoiding the virus through mitigation measures of mask wearing, hand and surface washing, and social distancing. These mitigation measures are straightforward and simple to apply, even though they have not been accepted throughout the United States.

Climate Change is far more complicated, occurring over decades instead of the two- to fourteen-day period between viral contagion and illness or the two or three years of the COVID-19 pandemic. Also, it is possible to confirm the presence of SARS-CoV-2 by testing for it. Climate Change has indirect effects that require acceptance of a scientific theory or paradigm before its effects can be attributed to it as a general cause. There are two parts to this paradigm. First, the climate is changing; second, global weather is getting warmer in specific episodes. And then people have to believe that global warming is caused by human consumption that results in trapped CO_2 in the Earth's atmosphere. Tests can be administered to conclusively determine the presence of SARS-CoV-2. But no isolated change in temperature, storm strength, or rise in water level is sufficient to prove or disprove the reality of Climate Change. According to relevant experts, SARS-CoV-2 is a distinct virus, but Climate Change is a long-term, irregular weather pattern over the entire planet Earth. One has to conceive of the planet having a general climate that is subject to change. Imagination is required to accept the reality of Climate Change.

Prevention entails avoiding an event, and with COVID-19 it could have been avoidance of the whole pandemic. Once the pandemic was under way, only mitigation has been possible. But mitigation depends on individual action such as wearing masks, practicing social distancing, or eventually getting vaccinated. In the early months of the COVID-19 pandemic, such mitigation was advised, sometimes strongly, by government officials, but enforcement has been patchy and reluctant. This situation is understandable, because forcing these measures on individuals against their will does constitute a violation of individual freedom and security.

Climate Change, by contrast, can only be addressed centrally, by government and business corporations, because individual and organization consumers do not produce their own fossil fuel products or build their own methane-producing factory farms. If certain products are no longer available to purchase or are too expensive, some will not consume them at all, and others will consume less of them. The individual choice here is simply the choice of the marketplace, where consumers do not control what is for sale. There are few mitigation measures for Climate Change that can be undertaken by individuals, and even these actions, such as avoiding development and construction in areas likely to be flooded by extreme storms or rises in sea level, require prior government regulation to become widespread.

Bottom-up mitigations of Climate Change undertaken by individuals are unlikely to amount to more than rhetorical gestures and superficial lifestyle changes (e.g., making compost, reducing travel, or recycling) that may or may not prompt top-down responses in the form of government programs and regulations and corporate retooling. The lifestyle changes are not superficial for the individuals making them—many are passionate in reducing their own carbon footprints, and their positions on Climate Change are part of their identities—but they are ineffective in redirecting or stabilizing the overarching process of Climate Change. As mentioned earlier (chapter 2), people have rights to free speech and expression, but they do not have the right to tell elected officials what to do.

Nevertheless, despite their differences, connections and similarities can be drawn between COVID-19 and Climate Change. Disaster ethics is relevant to both situations. In addition, the relative simplicity of the COVID-19 pandemic means that lessons can be learned from it, to apply to future zoonotic pandemics and maybe to Climate Change as well. The first section of this chapter is about disaster ethics and preparation, from a general perspective. Ethical issues pertaining to COVID-19 and Climate Change are then taken up, separately.

DISASTER ETHICS GENERALLY

Ethics is about choices and decisions that affect human life and well-being. Before and during a disaster, decisions and choices are made that affect human life and well-being, which means that these are ethical decisions and choices. But such decisions and choices are not often labeled ethical or moral decisions, except to justify them as the right thing to plan to do or to actually do. Also, and just as perplexing, there is a confusion between whether a decision or a choice is a moral matter, which entails that it may be either a morally right or a morally wrong decision or choice, and whether it is the right decision or choice. This is a confusion between the category and the right decision or choice concerning something within that category. Because decision makers know that they are dealing with ethical or moral matters, they simply assume that what they decide is the morally right thing. Their assumption that they are making the morally right decisions is understandable, but rarely is a specific code of ethics spelled out or referred to.

An example of conflating the category of moral decisions with the right moral decision has occurred in plans for COVID-19 triage where some are intended to receive priority in the allocation of a scarce resource, without moral justification of any depth (see chapter 4). Before then, during anticipation of a flu pandemic in 2007, the CDC offered guidelines that simply asserted the necessity for a shift from normal ethical considerations to the idea of the good of society, which included allocation of resources according to a ranking of social worth. Here is an excerpt from the CDC's "Ethical Guidelines in Pandemic Influenza":

> In ordinary circumstances, the distribution criterion, "to each according to his or her social worth," is not morally acceptable. However, in planning for a pandemic where the primary objective is to preserve the function of society, it is necessary to identify certain individuals and groups of persons as "key" to the preservation of society and to accord to them a high priority for the distribution of certain goods such as vaccines and antiviral drugs. Identification of key individuals for this purpose must be recognized for what it is: it is a social worth criterion and its use is justified in these limited circumstances.
>
> Among the goods that must be allocated is the time of health care professionals. It may be necessary to delegate the responsibility and authority to perform procedures and interventions customarily carried out by certain professionals to other individuals. For example, physicians may need to delegate duties to nurses, physicians' trained assistants.[4]

According to the CDC in the foregoing, it becomes ethical in a disaster to distribute treatment based on social worth. However, this is unfair, and simply calling it "ethical" does not make it so. The implicit assumption is that there are not enough materials and personnel to treat everyone, which would be fair. If disaster is not being (covertly and cynically) used as an excuse to rank people according to their "social worth," the background scarcity is a matter of prior preparation, as we shall soon see. Here, it is important to note that no justification was given for the "social worth criterion" and no definition of what it means to "preserve the function of society" was provided. If society has a function, it would presumably be a function for everyone, not only those of "social worth." What, then, is disaster ethics, or how might those who are interested think about it?

Disaster ethics is the application of existing ethical or moral systems or rules, or new ones that seem right in or for a crisis. For the theorist, there are two main ethical approaches: Deontology, or Duty Ethics; and Consequentialism, or Utilitarianism. Deontology (or Duty Ethics) has an abstract philosophical foundation based on Immanuel Kant's Categorical Imperative, and it has a Humanistic foundation that is more accessible. Kant's Categorical Imperative is an absolute rule of reason arrived at by imagining that all rational beings in the moral universe would or would not do the same thing contemplated. It was supposed to be a satisfactory answer to the question "What would happen if everybody did this?" The Humanistic formulation says, simply, "Don't use people!" or "No one is expendable." Both formulations result in moral actions that are obligatory or immoral actions that are prohibited, such as "You must do this" and "You must not do that." The moral activity in Deontology centers on values and intentions, held and formed before acting, and the consequences of the action taken are irrelevant to its moral goodness or badness. Everything is decided before the fact by a form of reasoning that is supposed to be the antithesis of instrumental reasoning, such as "Do this, in order to get that." Some of our highest principles are intuitively deontological (for instance, don't harm others; take care of children; be fair).[5]

Consequentialism is the general form of Utilitarianism that is usually attributed to Jeremy Bentham and John Stuart Mill. Both philosophers wrote with an audience of government leaders in mind. Utilitarianism is the more narrow theory developed by Bentham and Mill that the greatest amount of pleasure or happiness and the least amount of pain, for the greatest number of people, is the ultimate moral goal. Everyone is to count as one and no one more than one. Consequentialism is the broader version of this moral theory, according to which actions are morally good or bad, depending on their consequences.

In any emergency, it makes sense, ethically, to save as many as can be saved, given limitations of personnel and materials. Also, without a prior rescue plan, rescuers will just be ordered onto a scene to do the best they can. This is roughly based on consequentialist reasoning, and an emergency means that something must be done immediately. Left out here are deontological considerations that all of those who could be saved, should be saved. The deontological considerations can be given their due if there is adequate preparation beforehand.

Deontological reasoning was implicit in news reports that fewer Americans would have died from COVID-19 had there been better preparation before cases surged. In this case, since there were no antivirals or vaccines with which to respond or prepare, earlier mitigation measures of imposed or advised quarantines would have counted as preparation.[6] The general idea behind preparation is anticipation. If a disaster is anticipated before it occurs, it becomes a moral imperative to prepare for it. Preparation is the right thing to do, because it will save lives and preserve well-being. And preparation must be done, because if it is not done, more lives and well-being will be lost than if it is done. Preparation allows for fulfillment of both deontological principles that place a value on each and every human's life and well-being, as well as consequentialist principles that save or spare the greatest number.[7] Ideally, the greatest number becomes everyone who can be saved.

THE ETHICS OF COVID-19

The gap between what should be done in ethical or moral terms, which includes both preparation and mitigation, and what is done in reality has to be accepted as a problem that is sometimes intractable—although it is necessary to think about closing this gap as best as can be done. Education and self-interest could work to close this gap. Many ethical issues are single events, but a pandemic is a series of events over an unknown period of time, which requires both preparation at different stages and ongoing mitigation. In disaster, as for other unwanted kinds of events that allow the insurance industry to thrive, prudence can and should come into play. Preparation for COVID-19 was inadequate before the pandemic got under way, and mitigation (e.g., mask wearing and social distancing) therefore became even more important and urgent as the pandemic progressed. At every stage of the pandemic, preparation for the next anticipated stage is still possible. The development of vaccines is, for example, a form of preparation. Once the importance of preparation and mitigation, both before the entire event and during its progression, is understood, not preparing becomes a dereliction of duty that is morally reprehensible, instead of merely not doing something.

The politicization of COVID-19 mitigation needs to be addressed as part of the moral gap between what ought to be done and what ought not to be done. That is, the pandemic ought to have been prepared for, and then, failing that, mitigated. The politicization of mitigation is something that ought not to have been done, because it has distracted many from what they ought to do to mitigate the pandemic. As a result, many people simply do need more "granular" information about what they stand to lose from acceptance of risk and non-mitigation, as well as what they might gain from it.

Many have made it a matter of their individual constitutional rights to not wear a mask. This is the Red state–Blue state conflict already discussed in chapter 2: the division of individual action in a pandemic along Democratic and Republican party lines. The question then becomes whether people will give up a political position that brings them no real benefit and instead real harm, if not before they are harmed, then after. Maureen Dowd put it very well in a *New York Times* column about government officials who have become ill or died from contracting COVID-19 after refusing to wear face masks: "So conservatives are willing to embrace a new ethos? Give me liberty. And death."[8]

The individual-rights issue has been so easily countered that it should not require reiteration. Concerned citizens and celebrities have been shouting it on the airways since early spring 2020: "I may have a right to risk infection myself, but if I am already infected, I do not have a right to infect you against your will. And I may not know whether I am infected, because some percentage of all COVID-19 cases are asymptomatic."[9] Therefore, the obligation to wear a mask trumps the individual right not to wear a mask. Ethically, this reasoning has roots in natural law principles that we may not harm one another. Politically, it is a limit on rights in exceptional circumstances, for the sake of "the public good." Or it may be that the right not to wear a mask is canceled by the right of someone else not to be infected. At any rate, this ethical and political issue surrounding mask wearing is not new to COVID-19. It harkens back to the 1918 Spanish Flu pandemic, when there were public protests by unmasked people, many of whom were subsequently fined or arrested (e.g., for spitting on the street, refusing to wear masks, or smoking cigars through holes in their masks).[10]

Such struggles over mitigation would not have been necessary with adequate preparation beforehand. The main lesson that could be learned from COVID-19 would be that it is important to prepare for the next pandemic. Already on the horizon is a zoonotic virus with small outbreaks in humans and pigs, which is currently under surveillance. On July 2, 2020, the CDC reported studies under way since 2016 of "G4" Eurasian (EA) avian-like H1N1 viruses in pigs in China. These viruses are able to infect human beings and are spread through respiratory droplets. While three human infections were confirmed, 10 percent of swine workers showed evidence of prior infection after blood samples were taken. It is not known whether these "G4" viruses are contagious from person to person.[11] However, it took a while to determine the human-to-human transmissibility of SARS-CoV-2, and the physics of its aerosols and contagion through them remains inconclusive.[12] Therefore, should the G4 viruses spread, there is reason to be concerned that they might result in a future pandemic.

The G4 viruses are not unique. There is a broad solution that could "virus-proof the planet" as a prudent course of preparation, as discussed in chapter 1. This form of preparation seems entirely called for given the disruption caused by SARS-CoV-2, which has been partly the result of failures to heed earlier expert warning. In February 2018, a group convened by the World Health Organization (WHO) listed big public-health-risk diseases for which there were no conclusive remedies. Their list included Ebola, SARS, Zika, and Rift Valley fever, as well as "Disease X," a pathogen that would emerge from animals in a place where there was growing encroachment on natural habitats. Disease X would quickly spread and become a big pandemic that would "leave economic and social devastation in its wake." COVID-19 is Disease X! And as yet, there are no credible defenses against Disease Y or Disease Z.

Peter Daszak, a disease ecologist who heads EcoHealth Alliance, has proposed with colleagues a worldwide effort to find and track hundreds of thousands of unknown pathogens that could become future pandemics. Blood samples of people living in places where they might break out would be taken, and data collected would be used to develop drugs and vaccines before such diseases became outbreaks. Viruses are the cause of over two-thirds of new human diseases. Viruses evolve rapidly and can thereby adapt to new hosts. (These routes were followed by HIV-1 [the AIDS virus] that originated in chimpanzees and SARS-CoV-1, which began in bats, the presumptive origin of SARS-CoV-2 as well.) The proposed Global Virome Project would identify millions of unknown viruses and map their genomes, which can now be done very inexpensively. The total cost would be about $4 billion, and 70 percent of it could be done for $1.5 billion (which seems cheap, but even a cost of $10 billion yearly would still be cheap). So far, this is a project in need of funding. A Global Immunological Observatory could monitor blood banks and discarded medical blood samples for new viruses, particularly those in bats. (There is a scientific consensus that bat colonies are reservoirs of viruses that live in humans, and the area of Laos, Myanmar, Vietnam, and parts of south and southwest China has been identified as a hot spot.)[13]

The general idea of developing broad-spectrum antivirals and vaccines has been validated through the success of Remdesivir in treating COVID-19, although it was originally developed as a treatment for Ebola.[14] Remdesivir is an example of inadvertent preparation. A number of more deliberate preparations for COVID-19 could have been undertaken. Identifying who should have done what is not a matter of blame, although there is that, but experience from which future approaches can be learned. The preparation that would have had an impact in COVID-19 included some selective attention to warnings during the early phases of the pandemic, so that life-saving mitigation could have begun earlier under the Stafford Act (see chapter 2). More important than that, a general attitude of readiness for a pandemic could have been in place beforehand. In March 2020, *Politico* directed public attention to a sixty-nine-page National Security Council guidebook from the Obama administration that was at the disposal of the Trump administration. This text was developed in 2016, to assist leaders "in coordinating a complex U.S. Government response to a high-consequence emerging disease threat anywhere in the world."

The "Playbook for Early Response to High-Consequence Emerging Infectious Disease Threats and Biological Incidents" outlined questions to ask, who should be asked, and the kinds of decisions that would be necessary. (There is no evidence that the Trump administration was aware of the playbook or would have been interested in it if they were.)[15] Medicines and supplies for a pandemic would have been kept in the Strategic National Stockpile. However, by early March 2020, when COVID-19 was barely under way, it was already doubtful that demand by states could be met from this national resource.[16] To sum up, adequate preparation for a pandemic would require anticipation in prior federal government planning and material stockpiling, neither of which were in order before COVID-19, or even after it was under way.

THE ETHICS OF CLIMATE CHANGE

Both the COVID-19 pandemic and Climate Change share human activity as causes. Those who in one way or another deny either or both share an oblivion about the nature of Homo sapiens life on the planet. But despite conspiracy theories about its origin, the mechanism of COVID-19 contagion and how it affects the human body are not difficult to understand, because everything about it takes place within human society. Disease is part of society. Moreover, as individuals, we already understand diseases and somewhat understand diseases that can be caught from animals, which are life-forms we also understand. Climate Change is more difficult to understand on a fundamental level, because it requires thinking outside of society, in much bigger physical terms.

We need to think about the Earth's atmosphere that separates us from "space." This is not easy for many to do at this time, not least because there has not been a humanized space program for a number of years. On August 2, 2020, two astronauts made the first splashdown reentry in forty-five years. This involved getting their craft out of orbit and racing through the Earth's atmosphere at speeds causing 3,500-degree Fahrenheit heat to the outside of their capsule. They reported very loud noises en route, which sounded like animal groans and roars, rather than machinery. This whole *Crew Dragon* adventure, undertaken by SpaceX and NASA, should have galvanized national attention, but it passed like a blip amid pandemic and political news reports. It was reported, but not re-reported and analyzed the way our current overriding preoccupations are.[17] We have to develop an understanding of something beyond weather that is the cause of weather as we experience it, and that is climate. Climate occurs within the atmosphere of Earth.

The mechanism of global warming is simple enough to be taught in middle school. The Earth gets light and heat from the sun and also radiates heat (infrared radiation). Some gases in the Earth's atmosphere, such as oxygen, are transparent, so light and heat can pass through them. Other gases—greenhouse gases (GHG)—retain heat that is radiated from the Earth, and they reflect that heat back to Earth. GHG include carbon dioxide (CO_2), methane (CH_4), nitrous oxide (N_2O), and fluorinated gases. Excessive amounts of these gases are the cause of what is called "global warming," a rise in average Earth temperatures that is some amount beyond preindustrial global temperatures.[18] About 80 percent of global warming is believed to be caused by CO_2 from fossil fuel use, and about 17 percent is from animal agriculture fertilizers (N_2O) and gases (CH_4).[19] However, the existential meaning of global warming does not lie in temperature percentages or chemical compounds but in the experience of changes in weather and the environment that have substantial effects on the quality of human life.

Modern humans live in societies of human construction. Society in any case is an interlocking system of systems of human relationships and the exchanges of physical things. Except for extraordinary circumstances of isolation, human beings cannot get out of society. Even the most adventurous excursions into the wild refer back to society; the most intact pre-contact indigenous groups cannot escape the incursions of society. Within society, which is to say, the world as humans experience it, physical things are exchanged among humans and passed from humans to the environment outside of society, while other things, such as weather, go in. In going into society, material becomes societized (for instance, infrared radiation becomes heat that affects human beings in their societal activities). The natural environment is thus a source of physical things, some of which are necessary for bare human life, such as air and water, although even these are to some extent purified or their temperature changed. What humans do with the physical things within society has effects on physical things in the natural environment outside of society.

Understanding the basic economy between humans in society and the natural environment outside of society requires an ability to accept that wanting or needing something is no guarantee of getting it. This is a matter of accepting limits, an ethical issue of character, in being able to reckon with reality that doesn't fulfill one's wishes. If humans fail to collectively develop the character necessary for recognizing and addressing the basic economics of societal-environmental exchanges, including natural limits, the collectivity is unlikely to survive. This means that surviving Climate Change is a moral matter, because human life and well-being are at stake, and decisions and choices can be made that will affect outcomes. It would be best (for us) if these moral issues can be resolved in favor of survival, peacefully, with compassion. But if conflict becomes intense in a context of extreme disaster, we could all perish from the combined destruction caused by human conflict and the natural disaster.

In *After Sustainability*, John Foster discusses three main forms of denial. In literal denial, people simply negate that something is happening (as, for instance, so many did for so long concerning Climate Change);[20] interpretative denial accepts that something is happening, but not in a way that affects the interpreter; implicative denial may accept the effects of something like Climate Change but evade what should be done as a result.[21] Implicative denial is the most interesting form of denial, because the hard work of persuasion and understanding has already been done and all that remains is the "last mile" between thought and action.

Another way of describing implicative denial would be to show how it violates Aristotle's practical syllogism that is supposed to conclude with concrete action.[22] Speech is not generally action, but talking to someone about a subject that one knows will not be well received often is. About three-quarters of those who now accept the reality of Climate Change, and believe it will have harmful effects on them, do not talk about it to family members and friends.[23] Further study would be necessary to uncover the reasons for this silence. This absence of communication is a form of implicative denial, because it is natural to discuss important, disturbing issues with family members and friends, and if the issue is important enough, it may be obligatory to do so. So this failure of communication not only denies the implications of one's beliefs but also is a failure to act in the face of discomfort, conflict, or embarrassment. We could say that those who are "in" implicative denial about Climate Change are informed but not activated. (The situation may be like someone who knows that smoking is generally harmful, and harmful to them personally, yet fails to quit.)

Another ancient Greek concept might be useful here: the idea of *akrasia* in the sense of weakness of will.[24] While mitigating against COVID-19 may have been irretrievably politicized for the time being, or until enough "influencers" get sick and die, the situation may be different concerning Climate Change. With Climate Change, the rhetorical bubble may not be as distracting or as impermeable as the political rhetoric that has paralyzed adequate disaster response in the case of COVID-19. The implicative denial of Climate Change and its subsequent akrasia is not so much an opposition to action to mitigate or forestall Climate Change, as it is more simply a failure to act, a failure of will to attend to fundamental necessities of survival. Such akrasia is a type of decadence, although not the kind of decadence that is a preoccupation with frivolities or an absence of new ideas, as, for instance, Ross Douthat recently claimed.[25]

Akrasia in an absence of public policy will was evident in conditions that contributed to raging forest fires throughout California, Oregon, and Washington during early September 2020. A full year's fire destruction occurred in a matter of three days in some places.[26] Environmentalists have warned for decades that temperature warming, flammable development too close to forest lands, and the practice of putting out fires and restoring vegetation all contribute to more destructive fires.[27] While comparatively less expensive housing in natural environments is in high demand, construction should be balanced against risk, and flame-retardant materials more extensively required. But so far, even the most vulnerable states and localities have not put such preparation into effect. And, nationally speaking, there is as yet no comprehensive program for mitigating or preparing for Climate Change. In the aftermath of record fires in California, Democrats lined up on sounding the alarm concerning Climate Change, while Republicans emphasized forest management.[28]

People already have ideas concerning action for Climate Change, principally that they ought to demand that their elected officials enact measures to restrict fossil fuel production and limit animal agriculture. This does not require giving up petroleum-fueled transportation and consuming only plant products for protein, but simply limiting the supply of petroleum fuels and animal protein. These would be political demands, because they are demands of government. The implicative denial of those who personally believe that Climate Change is a real problem, about which they are concerned but fail to discuss with family members and friends, is a lack of political activation. This lack plays out as a lack of character, but the failure of communication and aversion to conflict that might motivate it may indeed be genuine ignorance about how to activate oneself in accord with what one knows without discomfort or disloyalty.

Political activism is broadly understood to be a willingness to join certain causes and lend one's voice and body to petitions and protests in favor of the goals of those causes. Not everyone has the energy or inclination to do that, but it is only one part of political activism and all too often its effects may be merely rhetorical and expressive. Another (and perhaps more important) aspect or kind of political activism is, quite simply, informed voting. Public debates about voting focus on who has access to polls and gerrymandering, with an implicit understanding that one party tries to block those from voting who will vote for the candidates of the competing party. This is indeed a problem, but it is not the only problem with voting as it pertains to akrasia concerning the political activation of most who recognize the dangers of Climate Change but do not talk about it. Simply being able to vote and voting is not sufficient. Also required is being informed about the Climate Change commitments and agendas of political candidates and seeking out or demanding information about those agendas before voting.

Voting has built-in privacy. It is not necessary that people publicize informed voting for candidates who are committed to addressing Climate Change. They do not have to tell those with whom they do not discuss Climate Change about how they vote. Widespread pre-election polls and focus groups create a false impression that voting is a transparent act. It is transparent to those whose job it is to count and add up votes, but it is not transparent to everyone with whom the voter would otherwise converse.

COVID-19 AND CLIMATE CHANGE TOGETHER

What humans want and need from the natural physical environment may be unlimited, but the natural environment itself has limits. Nonhuman living things also have wants and needs, some in conflict with those of humans. The environment outside of society does not function unconditionally to supply human (or nonhuman) wants and needs. It merely functions or ceases to function in ways that may or may not supply human wants and needs. Zoonotic viral pandemics and Climate Change have occurred through human causes operating in oblivion to the functioning of the nonhuman environment. The overarching question is whether humans in society can collectively, broadly, and even popularly acquire enough knowledge of nonhuman environments to save themselves.

We should focus on specific environmental functioning in how the effects of global warming connect Climate Change with future pandemics. First, animals flee higher temperatures, and second, the global productive trajectory and population increase drive more intense human development. The result is that animals and their diseases are brought into closer contact with human beings. In addition, the same causes of Climate Change are health hazards that affect the same vulnerable populations who suffer most from pandemics such as COVID-19. At the same time, there are new economic burdens of failing to prepare by reducing the same pollutants from fossil fuel consumption that contribute to global warming. According to Aaron Bernstein, director of the Harvard T. H. Chan School of Public Health's Center for Climate, Health, and the Global Environment:

> When you look at this question purely from a financial standpoint, air pollution is a drag on economic growth and solutions to address have been enormously cost-effective in the United States. In 2011, a study by the Environmental Protection Agency that looked at the costs and benefits of the Clean Air Act found that every $1 invested to reduce air pollution returns up to $30 in benefits. The only thing our health and our economy can't afford is climate inaction.[29]

As with the numbers pertaining to global warming, the economic numbers do not adequately describe the quality of human illness and suffering. However, leaders know mainly how to address the problem of global warming economically. And the economic approach taken by government is, in our society, the lever for stasis and deterioration or mitigation and solution. Money spent—or not spent—is literally the bottom line. While funds allocated for COVID-19 response and ongoing preparation and mitigation are not in the same "lane" as funds allocated for Climate Change, it is unfortunate if COVID-19 spending is used as a justification for not preparing or mitigating for Climate Change.

For instance, the budgetary stress caused by COVID-19 mitigation in New York State was the reason Governor Cuomo gave for postponing the $3 billion Restore Mother Nature Bond Act that was intended to reduce flooding in vulnerable communities, restore wildlife habitat, and generally prepare for Climate Change.[30] There should not be a "race to the bottom" competition for desperate, worthy, public health programs. But if finite public money must be prioritized, then Climate Change might be viewed as the general problem, of which COVID-19 is a specific symptom.

On September 9, 2020, *Politico* and the *New York Times* gave accounts of a forthcoming report commissioned from a task force by a financial regulatory agency, the US Commodities Futures Trading Commission. The likelihood of increasing severe storms, floods, and fires accompanying changes in climate was projected to pose "serious emerging risks to the U.S. financial system," and regulators were advised to "move urgently and decisively." Projected damages were forecast to disrupt commodity markets, mortgage companies, and the insurance industry. Mitigation, including limits (caps) on fossil fuel use and taxes on oil companies, would require government controls, enacted either by Congress or by presidential order. Commentators did not anticipate such action by the Trump administration, but it was predicted that a Biden administration would have the political will to enact measures. The main problem in addressing Climate Change is its duration through episodes in different places over years. That spasmodic aspect of Climate Change–related weather events has had a parallel with different surges of COVID-19 in different geographical locales, and it remains to be seen whether disasters of this form can be recognized by enough leaders, and the public, to effectively mitigate them.[31]

CONCLUSION

Tragedy and Resilience

"Alice had got so much into the way of expecting nothing but out-of-the-way things to happen, that it seemed quite dull and stupid for life to go on in the common way."
—Lewis Carroll, *Alice's Adventures in Wonderland*

"The greatness of America lies not in being more enlightened than any other nation, but rather in her ability to repair her faults."
—Alexis de Tocqueville, *Democracy in America*

Our present disorder is a jumble of old ideas and structures together with anticipated disruptions, while some people demand new ideas. In this sense, there is an ongoing battle between the past and the present. The disorder in the United States has been discussed as the uneven response in a federal system. Along with that, or perhaps fitting neatly into it, has been a weakened federal government with a president attempting to function as a king. Aristotle's description of tragedy, as quoted in the first epigraph to this book, has so far been fulfilled. America is the hero, neither highly virtuous nor highly vicious, and overall respectable, with settled traits of character that lead to errors in judgment. The errors in judgment have resulted in a collective fall. It is the settled traits of—and within—the national character that have led to collective and individual errors of judgment, followed by illness, death, and disruption that could have been avoided with better judgment. This has all been the so-called X-ray effect of COVID-19, which finds us where we are and shows us to ourselves. However, the American tragedy goes further, because it is not the result of one error or destructive consequence, but rather many errors and consequences over the period of the pandemic in 2020.

One error of judgment can be just that—an error—but many errors add up to an ongoing rigidity of character. This pandemic and future disasters that unfold over time require changes in custom and character. This is what's known as *resilience*. More Americans will need to develop resilience for this tragedy to be over and future tragedies avoided. That there is a future is the distinction of a tragedy in a nation compared to a literary creation or performance, which, as art, is temporally contained. So long as a nation and its form of government continue in historical time, tragedy one year need not continue into the next year. The social-political crises of 2020 can be resolved in 2021.

The account in this book of the effects of the pandemic on different segments of American society has overall been grim, but it has been an organized account. If responses going forward are organized, we may not be happy as the book's Zen epigraph promises, but we may avoid a certain amount of misery. The US federal structure of national, state, and local government has not been fully equal to the present crisis, although failures of the federal government have been countervailed by rational and efficient reactions within some states and localities. Still, as it stands, no states have sufficient resources to completely address the present crisis on their own: they don't have the medical resources, they are running out of money, or they lack the resolve to practice necessary mitigation when there have been surges of the disease. Needed is a president with a resilient character, expressed in realistic problem solving, together with a legislature that is focused on the public good, instead of the political careers of those who make it up. Needed is professionalism in government, based on the realities of the problems faced by ultimate constituents—the people. This would be government by elected officials who understand the need for experts and freely have recourse to their views so that they can rationally base decisions on them, for the good of their constituents—the people. It would be evidence-based government, unencumbered by competing identities.[1] It can never be perfect, but it can avoid both political and societal disaster.

With such stability in government, future disasters and disruptions, especially new pandemics, might be met with better preparation. On October 21, 2020, the National Center for Disaster Preparedness at the Earth Institute of Columbia University reported that based on comparative analysis and the application of proportional mortality rates, between 130,000 and 210,000 COVID-19 deaths in the United States could have been avoided with adequate preparation.[2] (At the time of the report, over 210,000 deaths from COVID-19 was a widely circulated count.) In late June 2020, there was scientific concern about a virus detected in pigs and identified since 2016, which is believed to be capable of infecting humans and starting a new pandemic.[3] Indeed, the CDC has reported taking action to prepare against such G4 Swine Flu viruses when no cases had been detected in the United States.[4] It would be possible to "pandemic-proof" the planet, as discussed in chapter 10, but if past reactions to preparation are a guide, this is not likely to happen. We do not yet know whether there will be adequate preparation for future developments of COVID-19 in the United States.

However, the United States is not alone in pandemic limbo and failure. There is a worldwide reluctance to prepare for disaster. Part of this reluctance may be an inchoate understanding of Quarantelli's definition of disaster as the natural event *plus* the human reaction to it. There may be an implicit understanding that it is impossible to prepare for how human beings will react to future pandemics, climate change, or any other disaster. Survivalists prepare for literal natural disasters with bunkers holding medicine and supplies of food meant to last for many years. They may also have a supply of guns and ammunition, which is a pessimistic way of preparing for how others may react. That is the narrow, fearful approach. More broadly, and toward accepting new challenges, the reactions to disaster cannot be forecast, because they are dynamic creative processes, some opportunistic and selfish, but others fair and generous. Preparation is an ongoing process throughout the time period of a disaster. There are many opportunities for flexibility and the changes that constitute resilience.

There has been much talk about how the "new normal" will be different from what we are used to. The future is always different from what we are used to. It will probably be an impossible exercise in hypothetical reasoning to determine how things will be different without the COVID-19 pandemic. This won't stop pundits from such speculation, but the long view tells us that human societies have changed in drastic ways in the past and will likely do the same in the future. Instead of referring to a "new normal," it is more precise to think about a new reality, or just think about the future, what seems likely to happen and what could go wrong.

In *Pandemic!* (published in June 2020), Slavoj Žižek relates a joke about a man who orders coffee without cream. The waiter tells him that they do not have cream, only milk, and asks whether he would like coffee without milk. Žižek thinks that enforced solitude for those who work at home anyway and do not go out and about much is nonetheless a tribulation, because the nature of what is absent has changed.[5] John Locke made the same distinction in discussing liberty as the absence of external constraint, so that even if one wanted to remain in a room, being locked into it would be a loss of liberty.[6] If we get what we want, why should choice or compulsion make such a difference? Is it a simple matter of moral principle that we value our freedom and, with that, we want to know that we have the options not taken? Or is it because the reasons we tell ourselves for why we are in specific situations matter to us, and having chosen something means that we are responsible for it, whereas having it imposed upon us makes us passive or victimizes us?

There is a third explanation, which leaves out the milk or cream case, about the nature of what we do not have, but it is closer to Locke's example of being locked into a room one wanted to be in anyway. It's simply that our liberty—the force of choosing something and getting that thing, or deciding to act, and acting, without external obstacles—is important in and of itself. If disaster includes how we react to unwanted natural events, it is important that we feel we have choices in how to react. However, "ought implies can." We cannot freely choose something impossible or unlikely in the face of our best information.

COVID-19 has indeed been revelatory. Social inequalities and injustices have been revealed, as has the structure of US federalism and localism. Also revealed, through the realities of contagion, are the myriad ways in which human beings are physically connected. Normal connections become dangerous in a time of contagion. And the risk of contagion has intersected with ideas of personal liberty. Normally, one has the liberty to move about in public, get close to others as the situation requires, and choose how to present oneself. But the necessity for social distancing and mask wearing interdict that opportunity. Some

Americans have easily grasped the physical facts of contagion and cho-sen to mitigate against them. Others seem unable to reconcile their liberty with such mitigation, to the point of violent resistance.

Democracy is a concept. Everyone can grasp in a vague sense that it means government should benefit those governed, or else they would not consent or continue to consent to it. At stake in a time of crisis are different conceptions of democracy. Democracy can mean majority rule, protection of individual rights, inclusion of everyone in its stated scope, obedience to standing laws and traditions, or some combination of these four. The benefit of those governed can refer to literally every-one or select subgroups. In play during COVID-19 have been these different conceptions of democracy.

I finished most of this book about a week before Election Day 2020. I originally thought this update would comment on the results of the election. But now I don't think that matters. Whoever is the next US president, some of the people will develop resilience as COVID-19 progresses, and some won't. And in the few remaining days before the election, the tragedy is ongoing, not only in increased cases of infection and deaths but also in small episodes of disappointment and misery. Consider the following campaign event that took place on October 27, 2020.

After President Trump held a rally at a Nebraska airport Tuesday night, thousands of the president's supporters were left stranded for hours in plummeting temperatures. Seven people were reportedly tak-en to area hospitals with hypothermia; as of the time of writing, their condition is unclear.

Trump had finished his remarks at Eppley Airfield and flown away on Air Force One, at which point the rally crowd, which numbered about six thousand in total, was meant to be bused back to parking lots ringing the base—at least one of which was almost four miles away. But the buses meant to transport the attendees couldn't get through clogged one-way roads, so thousands were left standing and waiting.

Ambulances were called, and some wheelchair-bound attendees could not move because of the cold—it was about 10 degrees Fahren-heit.[7] Some doubtless caught the SARS-CoV-2 virus. By the time this book is published, some of them will likely have died from this collec-tion of risk and errors in judgment, including lack of planning and an apparent inability to change mind-sets. And at the end of this book, although not the end of the pandemic, it's appropriate to take a moment to reflect on such deaths that could so easily have been avoided.

POSTSCRIPT

A Primary Question about Democracy

Now, after the 2020 election, a few weeks before the end of the year, the tragedy continues. There are new surges of COVID-19 throughout the United States and European democracies. Safe and effective vaccines, developed on the cutting edge of biological engineering, are on the horizon. It is too soon to describe the success of these vaccines, their safety, or even their distribution. If vaccines wipe out COVID-19 as they have wiped out so many other infectious diseases, science and technology will have triumphed once more for the common good. But we are not there yet.

The aftermath of the 2020 US presidential election revealed how the government structure of American electoral democracy can survive a pandemic. Record numbers of people voted, election workers meticulously computed their votes, votes were certified, and electors became poised to vote for their states. This democratic process has carried on through onslaughts of baseless charges of fraud by the democratically defeated incumbent president.

However, the continuing surge in COVID-19 infections and deaths reveals a primary question about democracy: Given a gap between morality and practicality, on one side, and constitutional principles, on the other, should legal force be used to apply morality and practicality? It is now broadly understood that the new surges could have been curtailed if more people were willing to wear masks, avoid social gatherings, and defer traditional holiday celebrations. Those who are compliant with mitigation feel that they are on the right side concerning science. They also believe they are on the right side morally, because no one has the right to harm others, and we all have an obligation to take action to avoid such harm. It is thus considered morally wrong not to wear masks or practice appropriate social distancing and isolation during a pandemic. However, this moral perspective has not been uniformly persuasive.

Enter the primary question about democracy in our present context: How should those who are morally and practically wrong, but within their legal constitutional rights, be addressed? Although it is an imperfect and divided federal system, the United States is a democracy. This means that there is something that all citizens and residents are in together and to which they belong. In the political terms of democracy, moral right and wrong are supplanted by political necessities and pragmatics. It does not matter whether people who voted for the very flawed incumbent president were wrong. Their votes were still counted. And it does not matter whether those who refuse to wear masks and practice social distancing and isolation are morally wrong. They still have the right not to comply. It is important to acknowledge that their noncompliance is based on constitutional protections of freedom of assembly and personal privacy (i.e., the right not to wear a mask may be akin to a woman's right not to continue a pregnancy). They have a right to risk their own health and lives, and the question of what to do when exercise of that right poses a risk to the health and lives of others falls into a politically amorphous space.

This amorphous space is bounded on three sides in this pandemic, and how the boundaries shape the space can establish political customs and principles that go beyond the present pandemic. One side consists of the noncompliant, and we can assume that some number of them who survive will join others who refuse to get COVID-19 vaccines. A second side consists of those of us who are compliant with mitigation and probably likely to get vaccines. The third side is the government, on federal, state, and local levels.

We on the second side, and perhaps the new federal administration, as well as many state governments, will need to decide how much force and restriction to use to compel compliance with ongoing mitigation and available vaccination. Will there be fines? Imprisonment? Forced compliance? Will social institutions, companies, and organizations secure the right to require compliance with mitigation and vaccination for their members and employees to participate? It is us on the second side, the informed and morally concerned people in this democracy, who may have the ultimate say in what happens, because our side has won the 2020 presidential election—and that sets a tone. We could demand enforced compliance to be issued from the new federal and existing state governments or restrain our moral impulses and quiet our fears.

Compliance in the US federal system would not be easily accomplished without overwhelming force on federal and state levels. Enforcement will ultimately depend on local authorities, who may resist. States could call out the National Guard, and those states that refused to do that could be overridden by federal declarations of extreme emergency (including insurrection), which mobilized the US military. The result of this project is difficult to predict, but it would certainly create a structure that could be used against those of us who constitute a morally correct opposition in a different, future context. We may be the ones believed to be morally wrong, who pose a danger to others who call for government force to be used against us.

So here is another perspective on the present gap between morality and constitutionality. Preserve democratic—which is to say, in our case, constitutional—liberty as a good that is presently abstract for us but will likely be practical in the future. This would mean speaking and acting to protect the rights of those who, in exercising their rights, may harm us as well as themselves. But that is not all. The side that is morally correct and compliant in the COVID-19 pandemic needs to do more work to persuade and educate those who are morally incorrect and noncompliant. We should not "cancel" the opposition in this case, but rather strive to bring them into the commonality that is shared.

Naomi Zack
December 2020

NOTES

INTRODUCTION

1. This phrase, "from the middle of things," was suggested to me by Jon Sisk, now senior executive editor at Rowman & Littlefield, several years ago, as the title of an earlier book I was thinking of writing at the time, but which did not materialize in the way we discussed. The phrase itself is the title of J. S. Fletcher's 1922 novel, *The Middle of Things*. (The story is strangely absorbing, like Fletcher's other mysteries, consisting of a detailed account of a group effort in solving the puzzle of a crime. It has a happy ending. Fletcher was a "jigsaw epistemologist." All, or most, of these mysteries begin with protagonist confrontation with the brute fact of a murder in which perpetrator and motive are unknown. It should be added that some of these works contain anti-black and anti-Asian racial slurs and stereotypes, as well as vague anti-Semitism, which may surprise some readers, not unlike our present experience in real life.)

2. Alex Tabarrok, "A Pandemic Trust Fund," COVID Recovery Symposium, April 2020, https://www.thecgo.org/wp-content/uploads/2020/04/Pandemic-Trust-Fund.pdf.

I. THE VIRUS IN THE WORLD

1. William Wan, Carolyn Y. Johnson, and Joel Achenbach, "States Rushing to Reopen Are Likely Making a Deadly Error, Coronavirus Models and Experts Warn," *Washington Post*, April 22, 2020, https://www.washingtonpost.com/health/2020/04/22/reopening-america-states-coronavirus/.

2. Russell R. Dynes, "The Dialogue between Voltaire and Rousseau on the Lisbon Earthquake: The Emergence of a Social Science View," Disaster Research Center, 1999, citable URI: http://udspace.udel.edu/handle/19716/435.

3. John R. Mullin, "The Reconstruction of Lisbon Following the Earthquake of 1755: A Study in Despotic Planning," *Journal of the International History of City Planning Association* (1992): 45, https://scholarworks.umass.edu/larp_faculty_pubs/45.

4. Charles E. Fritz, "Disasters," in Robert K. Merton and Robert A. Nisbet, eds., *Contemporary Social Problems* (New York: Harcourt, 1961), 655.

5. NIM (National Institute of Medicine), "Disaster Health Information Sources: The Basics," Disaster Information, Management Resource Center, https://www.nlm.nih.gov/dis_courses/basics/01-000.html.

6. E. L. Quarantelli, "What Is Disaster? The Need for Clarification in Definition and Conceptualization in Research," Disaster Research Center, University of Delaware, Research, Series Report, Article 177 (1985): 41–73, citable URI http://udspace.udel.edu/handle/19716/1119.

7. Ibid., 47–48.

8. Ibid., 50.

9. Ibid., 48–49.

10. E. L. Quarantelli, P. Lagadec, A. Boin, "A Heuristic Approach to Future Disasters and Crises: New, Old, and In-Between Types," in E. L. Quarantelli, ed., *Handbook of Disaster Research*, Handbooks of Sociology and Social Research (New York: Springer, 2007).

11. Naomi Zack, "The Big Question with Naomi Zack," *Scientific Inquirer*, May 27, 2020, https://scientificinquirer.com/2020/05/27/the-big-question-with-naomi-zack-ethics-and-the-covid-19-pandemic/.

12. Thomas Nagel, "Moral Luck," in *Mortal Questions* (Cambridge, MA: Cambridge University Press, 1979), 24–38.

13. For examples, see William D. Cohan, "'People Will Die. People Do Die.' Wall Street Has Had Enough of the Lockdown," *Vanity Fair*, May 15, 2020, https://www.vanityfair.com/news/2020/05/wall-street-has-had-enough-of-the-lockdown; Sarah Newey, "'UNICEF Warns Lockdown Could Kill More Than COVID-19 as Model Predicts 1.2 Million Child Deaths.' Indiscriminate Lockdowns Are an Ineffective Way to Control COVID and Could Contribute to a 45 Per Cent Rise in Child Mortality," *Global Health Security Reporter*, *The Telegraph*, May 13, 2020, https://www.telegraph.co.uk/global-health/science-and-disease/unicef-warns-lockdown-could-kill-covid-19-model-predicts-12/; Fady Asly, "A Few of Us Might Die from COVID-19, but the Current Worldwide Lockdown Will Kill Many More People," *New Europe*, March 26, 2020, https://www.neweurope.eu/article/a-few-of-us-might-die-

from-covid-19-but-the-current-worldwide-lockdown-will-kill-many-more-people/.

14. David Hume, "Of Justice," in *An Inquiry Concerning the Principles of Morals* (Indianapolis, IN: Hackett, 1983), 22–23; also at *An Inquiry Concerning the Principles of Morals*, Project Gutenberg, Section III, "Of Justice," Part III, Justice, https://www.gutenberg.org/files/4320/4320-h/4320-h.htm.

15. Kai Nielsen, "Against Moral Conservativism," *Ethics* 82, no. 3 (1972): 219–31, https://www.journals.uchicago.edu/action/showCitFormats?doi=10.1086/291845.

16. See Bob Wallace, "Medical Innovations: From the 1918 Pandemic to a Flu Vaccine," National World War II Museum, April 13, 2020, https://www.nationalww2museum.org/war/articles/medical-innovations-1918-flu; M. Martini, N. L. Gazzaniga, N. L. Bragazzi, and I. Barberis, "The Spanish Influenza Pandemic: A Lesson from History 100 Years after 1918," *Journal of Preventive Medicine and Hygiene* 60, no. 1 (March 2019): E64–E67, published online March 29, 2019, DOI: 10.15167/24214248/jpmh2019.60.1.1205, https://www.ncbi.nlm.nih.gov/pmc/articles/PMC6477554/.

17. Greta Privitera, "Italian Doctors on Coronavirus Frontline Face Tough Calls on Whom to Save," *Politico.eu*, March 9, 2020, https://www.politico.eu/article/coronavirus-italy-doctors-tough-calls-survival/; see also the documentary "Inside Italy's War on COVID," *Frontline*, season 20, episode 19, PBS, March 19, 2020, https://www.pbs.org/wgbh/frontline/film/inside-italys-covid-war/.

18. For moral arguments for disaster preparation, see Naomi Zack, *Ethics for Disaster* (Lanham, MD: Rowman & Littlefield, 2009, 2010/2011); idem, "Ethics of Disaster Planning," *Philosophy of Management*, Special Issue, Ethics of Crisis, Per Sandin, ed., vol. 8, no. 2 (2009): 53–64; idem, "Philosophy and Disaster," *Homeland Security Affairs Journal*, vol. II, issue 1, article 5 (April 2006), https://www.hsaj.org/articles/176.

For calls for zoonotic viral pandemic preparation before COVID-19, see Ed Yong, "The Next Plague Is Coming: Is America Ready?" *The Atlantic*, July 2018, https://www.theatlantic.com/magazine/archive/2018/07/when-the-next-plague-hits/561734/; Matthew Mosk, "George W. Bush in 2005: 'If We Wait for a Pandemic to Appear, It Will Be Too Late to Prepare,'" ABC News, April 5, 2020, https://abcnews.go.com/Politics/george-bush-2005-wait-pandemic-late-prepare/story?id=69979013; see also David Quammen, "Why Weren't We Ready for the Coronavirus?" *New Yorker*, May 4, 2020, https://www.newyorker.com/magazine/2020/05/11/why-werent-we-ready-for-the-coronavirus.

19. Andrew Jacobs, "Grave Shortages of Protective Gear Flare Again as COVID Cases Surge," July 8, 2020, *New York Times*, https://www.nytimes.com/2020/07/08/health/coronavirus-masks-ppe-doc.html.

20. The precautionary principle is arguably a quagmire, depending on the context in which it is discussed and disputed. On the precautionary principle more widely, see *ScienceDirect*, "The Precautionary Principle," https://www.sciencedirect.com/topics/earth-and-planetary-sciences/precautionary-principle.

21. Lauren Egan, "Lysol Maker Warns against Internal Use of Disinfectants after Trump Comments," NBC News, April 24, 2020, https://www.nbcnews.com/politics/donald-trump/lysol-manufacturer-warns-against-internal-use-after-trump-comments-n1191586.

22. Robert Glatter, MD, "Calls to Poison Centers Spike after the President's Comments about Using Disinfectants to Treat Coronavirus," *Forbes*, April 25, 2020, https://www.forbes.com/sites/robertglatter/2020/04/25/calls-to-poison-centers-spike--after-the-presidents-comments-about-using-disinfectants-to-treat-coronavirus/#40984b501157.

23. Palli Thordarson, "The Coronavirus Is No Match for Plain, Old Soap—Here's the Science Behind It," *MarketWatch*, April 8, 2020, https://www.marketwatch.com/story/deadly-viruses-are-no-match-for-plain-old-soap-heres-the-science-behind-it-2020-03-08.

24. William A. Haseltine, "Which COVID-19 Antivirals Actually Work?" *Forbes*, May 11, 2020, https://www.forbes.com/sites/williamhaseltine/2020/05/11/which-covid-19-antivirals-actually-work/#37eacaac68c6.

25. For how the SARS-CoV-2 virus affects the human body, see Robin Marks, "Unveiling How Coronavirus Hijacks Our Cells to Help Rush New Drugs to Patients," UCSF News, March 25, 2020, https://www.ucsf.edu/news/2020/03/416986/unveiling-how-coronavirus-hijacks-our-cells-help-rush-new-drugs-patients; CDC, "About Novel Coronavirus (2019-nCoV)," US Centers for Disease Control and Prevention (CDC), February 11 2020, https://www.cdc.gov/coronavirus/2019-ncov/index.html; WebMD, "Coronavirus: What Happens When You Get Infected," https://www.webmd.com/lung/coronavirus-covid-19-affects-body#1.

26. See ibid.

27. Robert Preidt, *MedicineNet*, "Coronavirus Isn't Even 'Alive,' but Expert Explains How It Can Harm," https://www.medicinenet.com/script/main/art.asp?articlekey=229387 (undated, accessed July 7, 2020).

28. R. Lu, X. Zhao, J. Li, P. Niu, B. Yang, H. Wu, et al., "Genomic Characterisation and Epidemiology of 2019 Novel Coronavirus: Implications for Virus Origins and Receptor Binding," *The Lancet* 395, issue 10224 (February 2020): 565–74, DOI:10.1016/S0140-6736(20)30251-8. PMID 32007145.

29. Renhong Yan, Yuanyuan Zhang, Yaning Li, Lu Xia, Yingying Gou, Qiang Zhou, "Structural Basis for the Recognition of SARS-CoV-2 by Full-Length Human ACE2," *Science* 367, issue 6485 (March 27, 2020): 1444–48, https://

science.sciencemag.org/content/367/6485/1444, DOI: 10.1126/science.abb 2762.

30. Duke University Medical Center, "Evolution of Pandemic Coronavirus Outlines Path from Animals to Humans," *ScienceDaily*, www.sciencedaily. com/releases/2020/05/200529161221.htm (accessed July 8, 2020).

31. Malware, Norton, "What Is a Computer Virus?" https://us.norton.com/ internetsecurity-malware-what-is-a-computer-virus.html (accessed on July 7, 2020).

32. See *Computer Hope*, "Macro," https://www.computerhope.com/jargon/ m/macro.htm.

33. See Owen Covington, "How COVID-19 Is Similar to the Viruses Trying to Infect Your Computer," *Today at Elon*, Elon University, March 31, 2020, https://www.elon.edu/u/news/2020/03/31/how-covid-19-is-similar-to-the-viruses-trying-to-infect-your-computer/.

Professor of computer science Megan Squire at Elon University is here reported to have used the similarities in how to avoid infection between SARS-CoV-2 and computer viruses. She also discusses malware and ransomware as opportunistic exploitation of COVID-19. (I came across this article after having my own insight about the SARS-CoV-2 and computer virus similarities.)

34. Janet Levin, "Functionalism," *Stanford Encyclopedia of Philosophy* (Fall 2018), Edward N. Zalta (ed.), https://plato.stanford.edu/archives/fall2018/ entries/functionalism/.

35. Sophie Anderson, "Antivirus and Cybersecurity Statistics, Trends & Facts 2020," *Safety Detectives*, January 24, 2000, https://www.safetydetectives. com/blog/antivirus-statistics/.

36. *The Economist*, "Pandemic-Proofing the Planet," Science and Technology, June 25, 2020, https://www.economist.com/science-and-technology/2020/ 06/25/pandemic-proofing-the-planet.

2. FEDERALISM AND LOCALISM

1. See "The Nine Most Terrifying Words," YouTube, https://www.youtube. com/watch?v=xhYJS80MgYA.

2. Andrew Cuomo, https://www.brainyquote.com/quotes/andrew_cuomo_ 412750.

3. M. U. G. Kraemer, A. Sadilek, Q. Zhang, et al., "Mapping Global Variation in Human Mobility," *Nature Human Behaviour* (2020), https://doi.org/10. 1038/s41562-020-0875-0.

4. Matina Stevis-Gridneff, "E.U. Formalizes Reopening, Barring Travelers from U.S.," *New York Times*, June 30, 2020, https://www.nytimes.com/2020/06/30/world/europe/eu-reopening-blocks-us-travelers.html.

5. Maureen Callahan, "'We Should Blow Up the Bridges': Coronavirus Leads to Class Warfare in Hamptons," *New York Post*, March 19, 2020, https://nypost.com/2020/03/19/we-should-blow-up-the-bridges-coronavirus-leads-to-class-warfare-in-hamptons/.

6. Mark J. Rozell and Clyde Wilcox, *Federalism: A Very Short Introduction* (New York: Oxford University Press, 2019), 92–97.

7. See Kevin M. Wagner, "Layer Cake Federalism," Center for the Study of Federalism, https://encyclopedia.federalism.org/index.php/Layer_Cake_Federalism.

8. For some details regarding this history, see Kent Newmyer, "*John Marshall McCulloch v. Maryland* and the Southern States' Rights Tradition," 33 *John Marshall Law Review* 33, issue 4 (2000): 875–934.

9. See National Governors' Association (NGA), "Governors' Letter Regarding COVID-19 Aid Request," Executive Committee Letters NGA, April 21, 2020, https://www.nga.org/policy-communications/letters-nga/governors-letter-regarding-COVID-19-aid-request/. See also FEMA, "Overview of Stafford Act Support to States," https://www.fema.gov/pdf/emergency/nrf/nrf-stafford.pdf.

10. Matt Flegenheimer, "What Democracy Scholars Thought of Trump's Bible Photo Op," *New York Times*, June 2, 2020, https://www.nytimes.com/2020/06/02/us/politics/trump-holds-bible-photo.html.

11. Helene Cooper, "Milley Apologizes for Role in Trump Photo Op: 'I Should Not Have Been There,'" *New York Times*, June 11, 2020, https://www.nytimes.com/2020/06/11/us/politics/trump-milley-military-protests-lafayette-square.html.

12. Kyley Schultz, "Trump Orders National Guard Troops to Leave D.C.," *WUSA*, https://www.wusa9.com/article/news/local/dc/dc-troops-federal-out-of-washington-trump-orders-national-guard/65-0f7092d9-4756-4709-9632-b45df9a5c66b.

13. Matthew Daly/AP, "House Approves Bill to Make the District of Columbia the 51st State," *Time*, June 26, 2020, https://time.com/5860443/house-passes-dc-statehood-bill/.

14. Ronald Brownstein, "Red and Blue America Aren't Experiencing the Same Pandemic: The Disconnect Is Already Shaping, Even Distorting, the Nation's Response," *The Atlantic*, March 20, 2020, https://www.theatlantic.com/politics/archive/2020/03/how-republicans-and-democrats-think-about-coronavirus/608395/.

15. Ryan Lizza and Daniel Lippman, "Wearing a Mask Is for Smug Liberals. Refusing to Is for Reckless Republicans," Coronavirus, *Politico*, May 1, 2020, https://www.politico.com/news/2020/05/01/masks-politics-coronavirus-227765.

16. Stephen Groves and Dave Kolpack, "Dakotas Lead US in Virus Growth as Both Reject Mask Rules," Associated Press, September 12, 2020, https://apnews.com/f4988865f4fad739e099b17707f8727f.

17. For a comprehensive description of these federal directives and implements, see Emily Berman, "The Roles of the State and Federal Government in a Pandemic," *Journal of Nation Security Law and Policy* (2020), especially pages 4–8 out of 21; available at SSRN: https://ssrn.com/abstract=3617058 or http://dx.doi.org/10.2139/ssrn.3617058 (accessed June 27, 2020).

18. See Trisha Anderson, Frederic Levy, Michael Wagner, and Ryan Burnette, "State of Emergency: COVID-19, the Stafford Act, and What It All Means for Contractors," posted in "Coronavirus, COVID-19, Government Contracts Regulatory Compliance, State and Local Procurements," March 18, 2020, https://www.insidegovernmentcontracts.com/2020/03/state-of-emergency-COVID-19-the-stafford-act-and-what-it-all-means-for-contractors.

For the full legal version of the Stafford Act, see FEMA, Stafford Act, as Amended, and Related Authorities, FEMA P-592, May 2019, Homeland Security Act, as amended (Emergency Management-Related Provisions), https://www.fema.gov/pdf/emergency/nrf/nrf-stafford.pdf.

19. Donald J. Trump, "Letter from President Donald J. Trump on Emergency Determination under the Stafford Act," White House, Healthcare, issued on: March 13, 2020, https://www.whitehouse.gov/briefings-statements/letter-president-donald-j-trump-emergency-determination-stafford-act/; Charlotte Butash, "What's in Trump's National Emergency Announcement on COVID-19?" Biodefense, *Lawfare*, March 14, 2020, https://www.lawfareblog.com/whats-trumps-national-emergency-announcement-COVID-19.

20. Brittany De Lea, "Coronavirus Crisis: What to Know about the Stafford Act," FOXBusiness, March 25, 2020, https://www.foxbusiness.com/features/coronavirus-crisis-stafford-act.

21. See Brennan Center for Justice, "A Guide to Emergency Powers and Their Use," April 24, 2010, https://www.brennancenter.org/our-work/research-reports/guide-emergency-powers-and-their-use; Masha Simonova and Nathaniel Sobel, "Federal Executive Emergency Authorities to Address COVID-19," *Lawfare*, April 2, 2020, www.lawfareblog.com/federal-executive-emergency-authorities-address-COVID-19.

22. Libby Cathey, "Trump Now Calling Coronavirus Fight a 'War' with an 'Invisible Enemy,'" ABC News, March 17, 2020, https://abcnews.go.com/Politics/trump-coronavirus-task-force-economic-public-health-steps/story?id=

69646672; Zeke Miller, "Pence a Voice of Calm on Virus—Balancing Health, Politics," Federal News Network, April 24, 2020, https://federalnewsnetwork. com/government-news/2020/04/pence-a-voice-of-calm-on-virus-balancing-health-politics/.

23. For information on the CDC, see Joseph B. McCormick, MD, and Susan Fisher-Hoch, MD, *Level 4 Virus Hunters of the CDC: Tracking Ebola and the World's Deadliest Viruses* (Graymalkin Media, March 2020); Centers for Disease Control and Prevention (CDC), https://www.cdc.gov/; Eric Lipton, Abby Goodnough, Michael D. Shear, Megan Twohey, Apoorva Mandavilli, Sheri Fink, and Mark Walker, "The CDC Waited 'Its Entire Existence for This Moment'; What Went Wrong?" (consulted on June 25, 2020), *New York Times*, https://www.nytimes.com/2020/06/03/us/cdc-coronavirus.html.

24. Associated Press, *Washington Times*, October 1, 2002, "Records Reveal CDC Sent Germ Strains to Iraq in 1980s," https://www.washingtontimes.com/news/2002/oct/1/20021001-091445-2576r/. For sources on the other errors listed, see the notes in Wikipedia, "Centers for Disease Control and Prevention," https://en.wikipedia.org/wiki/Centers_for_Disease_Control_and_Prevention, June 14, 2020.

25. Michael D. Shear, "'They Let Us Down': 5 Takeaways on the C.D.C.'s Coronavirus Response," *New York Times*, June 3, 2020, https://www.nytimes.com/2020/06/03/us/cdc-virus-takeaways.html.

26. White House, Coronavirus Task Force, January 29, 2020, https://www.whitehouse.gov/briefings-statements/statement-press-secretary-regarding-presidents-coronavirus-task-force/.

27. Jemima McEvoy, "Reports: Trump Administration Pressured CDC to Change Asymptomatic Testing Guidelines," *Forbes*, August 26, 2020, https://www.forbes.com/sites/jemimamcevoy/2020/08/26/reports-trump-administration-pressured-cdc-to-change-asymptomatic-testing-guidelines/#61314b791f8b.

28. CDC, "Coronavirus Disease 2019 (COVID-19)," September 18, 2020, https://www.cdc.gov/coronavirus/2019-ncov/hcp/testing-overview.html.

29. Carl Zimmer and Noah Weiland, "In Reversal, White House Approves Stricter Guidelines for Vaccine Makers," *New York Times*, October 6/15, 2020, https://www.nytimes.com/2020/10/06/health/covid-vaccine-guidelines.html.

30. See Emergency Management Assistance Compact: The All Hazards National Mutual Aid System (EMAC), https://www.emacweb.org/.

31. For citations to relevant past cases, see Gibson Dunn, "The Constitutional Consequences of Governmental Responses to COVID-19: The Right to Travel and the Dormant Commerce Clause," May 1, 2020, https://www.gibsondunn.com/the-constitutional-consequences-of-governmental-responses-to-COVID-19-the-right-to-travel-and-the-dormant-commerce-clause/.

32. Ibid., from *New State Ice Co. v. Liebmann*, 285 U.S. 262, 311 (1932).

33. William Wan, Carolyn Y. Johnson, and Joel Achenbach, "States Rushing to Reopen Are Likely Making a Deadly Error, Coronavirus Models and Experts Warn," *Washington Post*, April 22, 2020, https://www.washingtonpost.com/health/2020/04/22/reopening-america-states-coronavirus/.

34. Joseph Spector, "Cuomo Rips Attempts to Ban New Yorkers' Travel to Other States, Vowing to Sue Rhode Island," lohud.com, New York State Team, March 28, 2020, https://www.lohud.com/story/news/politics/2020/03/28/cuomo-rips-possible-ban-new-yorkers-travel-vowing-sue-rhode-island/2934301001/.

35. New York State Government, "COVID-19 Travel Advisory," June 22, 2020, https://coronavirus.health.ny.gov/COVID-19-travel-advisory.

36. Amy Sherman, "Fact-Checking Jared Kushner's Comments on the National Stockpile," *PolitiFact*, Poynter Institute, April 3, 2020, https://www.politifact.com/article/2020/apr/03/fact-checking-jared-kushners-comments-national-sto/.

37. Jane C. Timm, "No Evidence for Trump's Suggestion That Masks Are 'Going Out the Back Door' of New York Hospitals," NBC News, March 30, 2020, https://www.nbcnews.com/politics/politics-news/no-evidence-trump-s-suggestion-masks-are-going-out-back-n1172251.

38. Jonathan Mahler, "A Governor on Her Own, with Everything at Stake," *New York Times Magazine*, June 27, 2020, https://www.nytimes.com/2020/06/25/magazine/gretchen-whitmer-coronavirus-michigan.html.

39. Abigail Censky, "The Boiling Resentment behind the Foiled Plan to Kidnap Gov. Whitmer," NPR, October 10, 2020, https://www.npr.org/2020/10/10/922610152/the-boiling-resentment-behind-the-foiled-plan-to-kidnap-gov-whitmer.

40. David A. Graham, "Governors Are Passing the Coronavirus Buck to Mayors," *The Atlantic*, June 18, 2020, https://www.theatlantic.com/ideas/archive/2020/06/covid-preemption-reversals/613210/.

41. Cassandra Pollock and Juan Pablo Garnham, "Texas City and County Leaders Ask Gov. Greg Abbott for Authority to Implement Local Stay-at-Home Orders," Coronavirus in Texas, *Texas Tribune*, June 29, 2020, https://www.texastribune.org/2020/06/29/texas-coronavirus-stay-at-home-harris-dallas/.

42. Conrad Nyamutata, "Do Civil Liberties Really Matter During Pandemics? Approaches to Coronavirus Disease (COVID-19)," *International Human Rights Law Review* 9, issue 1 (May 24, 2020): 62–98, https://brill.com/view/journals/hrlr/9/1/article-p62_62.xml.

43. Ruthann Robson, "Positive Constitutionalism in a Pandemic: Demanding Responsibility from the Trump Administration," *ConLawNOW* 12, issue 1 (2020): 15, https://ideaexchange.uakron.edu/conlawnow/vol12/iss1/2/.

44. Hallie Golden, Mike Baker, and Adam Goldman, "Suspect in Fatal Portland Shooting Is Killed by Officers during Arrest," *New York Times*, September 4, 2020, https://www.nytimes.com/2020/09/03/us/michael-reinoehl-arrest-portland-shooting.html.

45. Ashitha Nagesh, "Portland: How a 'Hyper-Liberal' City's Racist Past Is Resurfacing," BBC News, September 3, 2020, https://www.bbc.com/news/world-us-canada-53996159.

3. RHETORIC AND THE US CULTURE WARS

1. Schmoop.com, "Pay No Attention to that Man Behind the Curtain," Quotes, *Shmoop*, https://www.shmoop.com/quotes/pay-no-attention-man-behind-the-curtain.html.

2. Michael D. Shear, "Trump Retweets Racist Video Showing Supporter Yelling 'White Power,'" *New York Times*, June 28, 2020, https://www.nytimes.com/2020/06/28/us/politics/trump-white-power-video-racism.html.

3. Joseph E. Ledoux, "Cognitive-Emotional Interactions in the Brain," *Cognition and Emotion* 3, issue 4 (1989): 267–89, published online January 7, 2008, https://www.tandfonline.com/doi/abs/10.1080/02699938908412709.

4. See the text of former US secretary of defense General Jim Mattis's statement in response to this call for arms: Jim Mattis, "In Union There Is Strength," America Recons with Racial Injustice, NPR, June 4, 2020, http://www.npr.org/2020/06/04/869262728/read-the-full-statement-from-jim-mattis.

5. Bethania Palma, "Did Trump Say 'This Is a Great Day' for George Floyd?" *Snopes*, June 5, 2020, https://www.snopes.com/fact-check/trump-george-floyd-great-day/.

6. Jay Yarrow, "Peter Thiel Perfectly Summed Up Donald Trump in a Few Sentences," CNBC, November 9, 2016, https://www.cnbc.com/2016/11/09/peter-thiel-perfectly-summed-up-donald-trump-in-one-paragraph.html.

7. See CNN, "Reporter Asks Trump: What Do You Say to Scared Americans?" March 20, 2020, https://www.cnn.com/videos/politics/2020/03/20/trump-message-to-americans-coronavirus-presser-vpx.cnn.

8. Kaiser Health News (KHN), "Metrics-Focused Trump Laments Fact That Testing More People Means a Higher Case Count for U.S.," May 15, 2020, https://khn.org/morning-breakout/metrics-focused-trump-laments-fact-that-testing-more-people-means-a-higher-case-count-for-u-s/.

9. David Markowitz, "Trump Is Lying More Than Ever: Just Look at the Data," *Forbes*, May 5, 2020, https://www.forbes.com/sites/davidmarkowitz/2020/05/05/trump-is-lying-more-than-ever-just-look-at-the-data/#39b4e6ce1e17.

10. See Reuters, "Trump's Name to Be on Stimulus Checks Going to Americans: *Washington Post*," April 14, 2020, https://www.reuters.com/article/us-health-coronavirus-usa-checks/trumps-name-to-be-on-stimulus-checks-going-to-americans-washington-post-idUSKCN21X079; Donald G. McNeil Jr. and Andrew Jacobs, "Blaming China for Pandemic, Trump Says U.S. Will Leave the W.H.O.," *New York Times*, May 29, 2020, https://www.nytimes.com/2020/05/29/health/virus-who.html.

11. Mary L. Trump, PhD, *Too Much and Never Enough: How My Family Created the World's Most Dangerous Man* (New York, London: Simon & Schuster, 2020), 16, 17.

12. See *Encyclopedia Britannica*, "Royal Household of the United Kingdom," https://www.britannica.com/topic/Royal-Household-of-the-United-Kingdom.

13. Margaret Davies, "Home and State: Reflections on Metaphor and Practice," *Griffith Law Review* 23, issue 2 (2014): 153–75, DOI: 10.1080/10383441.2014.962447.

14. See Torin Monahan, "Securing the Homeland: Torture, Preparedness, and the Right to Let Die," *Social Justice* 33, no. 1 (2006): 95–105, https://publicsurveillance.com/papers/Securing_the_Homeland.pdf.

15. Esther Addley and Robert Booth, "Who Controls Whom? The Monarchy vs. the Media," *The Guardian*, November 8, 2016, https://www.theguardian.com/uk-news/2016/nov/08/who-controls-who-the-monarchy-v-the-media.

16. Rozina Sabur, "Trump Says He Had 'Automatic Chemistry' with the Queen as He Raves about Their Relationship," *The Telegraph*, June 7, 2019, https://www.telegraph.co.uk/news/2019/06/07/trump-says-had-automatic-chemistry-queen-raves-relationship/.

17. *Toofab* Staff, "Roseanne Barr Calls Donald Trump 'First Woman President' in Bizarre Video," Celebrity, *Toofab*, June 28, 2020, https://toofab.com/2020/06/26/roseanne-barr-calls-donald-trump-first-woman-president-in-bizarre-video/.

18. See "25th Amendment," Legal Information Institute, Cornell Law School, https://www.law.cornell.edu/constitution/amendmentxxv.

19. Sam Gringlas, "At Least 8 People Test Positive for Coronavirus after Rose Garden Event for Barrett," NPR News, October 3, 2020, https://www.npr.org/sections/latest-updates-trump-covid-19-results/2020/10/03/919851907/

at-least-7-people-test-positive-for-coronavirus-after-rose-garden-event-for-barr.

20. Frances Mulraney, "Full Transcript of Donald Trump's Address to the Nation from Walter Reed," *Daily Mail*, October 4, 2020, https://www.daily mail.co.uk/news/article-8802463/Full-transcript-Donald-Trumps-address-nation-Walter-Reed.html.

21. Ann Colwell, "Personal Loss, Pastoral Instincts and His Son's Rosary: What Defines Joe Biden," CNN Politics, August 21, 2020, https://www.cnn.com/2020/08/20/politics/borger-biden-documentary/index.html; see also "Joe Biden on Wearing His Son Beau's Rosary Beads: It's My Connection to Him," *Today*, November 13, 2020, https://www.youtube.com/watch?v=72oO7R0 CxSo.

22. Tamara Keith, Scott Detrow, Asma Kalid, and Mara Liasson, "'An Ally of the Light': Joe Biden Pledges Return to Hope and Compassion," *The NPR Politics Podcast*, August 21, 2020, https://www.npr.org/2020/08/21/904557510/an-ally-of-the-light-joe-biden-pledges-return-to-hope-and-compassion.

23. Bob Woodward, *Rage* (New York: Simon & Schuster, 2020).

24. Joshua Barbosa et al., "Outcomes of Hydroxychloroquine in Hospitalized Patients with COVID-19: A Quasi-Randomized Comparative Study," submitted to *New England Journal of Medicine*, Scholar One, June 15, 2020, https://www.sefq.es/_pdfs/NEJM_Hydroxychlorquine.pdf.

25. Michael Collins and David Jackson, "Tickets for Trump Campaign Rally Include Liability Disclaimer about Possible Exposure to Coronavirus," *USA Today*, June 11, 2020, https://www.usatoday.com/story/news/politics/2020/06/11/coronavirus-tickets-donald-trump-rally-include-liability-waiver/533488 5002/.

26. Taylor Lorenz, Kellen Browning, and Sheera Frenkel, "TikTok Teens and K-Pop Fans Say They Sank Trump Rally," *New York Times*, July 21, 2020, https://www.nytimes.com/2020/06/21/style/tiktok-trump-rally-tulsa.html.

27. Giovanni Russonello, "Trump's Tulsa Rally Attendance: 6,200, Fire Dept. Says," *New York Times*, June 22, 2020, https://www.nytimes.com/2020/06/22/us/politics/trump-rally-coronavirus.html.

28. Zolan Kanno-Youngs, Jennifer Steinhauer, and Kenneth P. Vogel, "Mayor Muriel E. Bowser of Washington, D.C., Dedicated an Area near the White House as Black Lives Matter Plaza on Friday," *New York Times*, June 5, 2020, https://www.nytimes.com/2020/06/05/us/politics/muriel-bowser-trump.html.

29. I am not going to specifically reference all or even a few of the hundreds of public references to the history of black oppression and who made them. Suffice it to note that Bill Moyer said that the murder of George Floyd was a lynching that the whole world witnessed, and Michelle Alexander's 2011 book,

The New Jim Crow: Mass Incarceration in the Age of Color Blindness, has been frequently invoked. Alexander's major theme is that the civil rights legislation was immediately met with racist backlash while at the same time the formal equality provided by that legislation sustained a fiction of color blindness. We can say that fiction has now been broadly discarded. For Bill Moyer's interpretation, see his June 9, 2020, interview with Christiane Amanpour, https://www.facebook.com/watch/?v=591136778198944.

30. For specifics on this federal aid, see Senator Ron Wyden's Office, "Summary of COVID-19 Bills and Available Resources," https://www.wyden.senate.gov/imo/media/doc/Summary%20of%20COVID-19%20bills%20and%20Available%20Resources%20(2).pdf.

31. Scott Neuman, "Medical Examiner's Autopsy Reveals George Floyd Had Positive Test for Coronavirus," June 4, 2020, NPR, https://www.npr.org/sections/live-updates-protests-for-racial-justice/2020/06/04/869278494/medical-examiners-autopsy-reveals-george-floyd-had-positive-test-for-coronavirus.

32. See P. Slovic, "'If I Look at the Mass I Will Never Act': Psychic Numbing and Genocide," *Judgment and Decision Making* 2, no. 2 (2007): 79–95, available at www.decisionresearch.org; P. Slovic, M. Finucane, E. Peters, and D. MacGregor, "The Affect Heuristic," in T. Gilovich, D. Griffin, and D. Kahneman, eds., *Intuitive Judgement: Heuristics and Biases* (Cambridge: Cambridge University Press, 2002).

33. See Michael Wines, "'Looting' Comment from Trump Dates Back to Racial Unrest of the 1960s," *New York Times*, May 29, 2020, https://www.nytimes.com/2020/05/29/us/looting-starts-shooting-starts.html.

34. See Nick Robins-Early, "The Violent Extremist Threat That's Growing during Nationwide Protests," Politics, *Huff Post*, June 12, 2020, https://www.huffpost.com/entry/boogaloo-protests-antifa-far-right_n_5ee3f503c5b6d5d0fc68f37d.

35. Jack Healy and Nicholas Bogel-Burroughs, "Calls for Transforming Police Run into Realities of Governing in Minnesota," *New York Times*, June 12, 2020, https://www.nytimes.com/2020/06/12/us/minneapolis-police-defunding.html.

36. Luis Ferré-Sadurní and Jesse McKinley, "N.Y. Bans Chokeholds and Approves Other Measures to Restrict Police," *New York Times*, June 12, 2020, https://www.nytimes.com/2020/06/12/nyregion/50a-repeal-police-floyd.html.

37. Amy Harmon and Sabrina Tavernise, "One Big Difference about George Floyd Protests: Many White Faces," *New York Times*, June 12, 2020, https://www.nytimes.com/2020/06/12/us/george-floyd-white-protesters.html.

38. See David Hessekiel, "Companies Taking a Public Stand in the Wake of George Floyd's Death," *Forbes*, June 6, 2020, https://www.forbes.com/sites/

davidhessekiel/2020/06/04/companies-taking-a-public-stand-in-the-wake-of-george-floyds-death/#1f5d36377214; Eden Stiffman, "Statements about George Floyd Are a Start, but How Will Organizations Live Their Values?" *Chronicle of Philanthropy*, June 9, 2020, https://www.philanthropy.com/article/Statements-About-George-Floyd/248953.

39. Jacques Maritain, "The Grounds for an International Declaration of Human Rights" (1947), in Micheline R. Ishay, ed., *The Human Rights Reader* (New York: Routledge, 2007), 2–6 (UDHR is reprinted in Ishay, 493–96).

40. See Naomi Zack, *Applicative Justice: A Pragmatic Empirical Approach to Racial Injustice* (Lanham, MD: Rowman & Littlefield, 2016), 65–88; Issues, United Nations Human Rights, Office of the High Commissioner, https://www.ohchr.org/EN/ProfessionalInterest/Pages/UniversalHumanRights Instruments.aspx.

41. See Ask Dag, "How Is the United Nations Responding to the Novel Coronavirus (2019-nCoV)/COVID-19 Outbreak?" Dag Hammarskjöld Library, https://ask.un.org/faq/281723 (consulted on July 2, 2020).

42. Mariel Padilla, "Who's Wearing a Mask? Women, Democrats and City Dwellers," *New York Times*, June 2, 2020, https://www.nytimes.com/2020/06/02/health/coronavirus-face-masks-surveys.html.

43. Julie Bosman, "Amid Virus Surge, Republicans Abruptly Urge Masks Despite Trump's Resistance," *New York Times*, July 2, 2020, https://www.nytimes.com/2020/07/01/us/coronavirus-masks.html.

44. Paul Best, "Trump 'All for Masks,' Looked like 'Lone Ranger' in One," Fox News, Business, Lifestyle, July 1, 2020, https://www.foxbusiness.com/lifestyle/trump-all-for-masks-looked-like-lone-ranger-in-one.

45. *CBS This Morning*, YouTube, "Trump Defends Monuments in Fiery Mt. Rushmore Speech," https://www.youtube.com/watch?v=QQOErcg_ask.

46. Larry Buchanan, Quoctrung Bui, and Jugal K. Patel, "Black Lives Matter May Be the Largest Movement in U.S. History," *New York Times*, July 3, 2020, https://www.nytimes.com/interactive/2020/07/03/us/george-floyd-protests-crowd-size.html.

47. See Naomi Zack, *Progressive Anonymity: From Identity Politics to Evidence-Based Government* (Lanham, MD: Rowman & Littlefield, 2020), especially chapters 3, 4, and conclusion.

4. INEQUALITY AND MARGINALIZATION

1. Clyde W. Yancy, MD, "COVID-19 and African Americans," *JAMA Network*, March 19, 2020, https://jamanetwork.com/journals/jama/fullarticle/2764789.

2. Quoted in Adam Harris, "It Pays to Be Rich during a Pandemic: How the Wealthy, Powerful and Connected Are Exploiting the Loopholes in Our Health Care System," *The Atlantic*, March 15, 2020, https://www.theatlantic.com/politics/archive/2020/03/coronavirus-testing-rich-people/608062/.

3. New York Region, *New York Times*, Andrew Cuomo Daily Briefing, "Cuomo Calls Subway Cars Filled with Homeless People 'Disgusting,'" April 4, 2020, https://www.nytimes.com/2020/04/28/nyregion/coronavirus-new-york-update.html#link-6eaeaa4a.

4. For more extensive discussions of these racisms, see Naomi Zack, ed., *Oxford Handbook of Philosophy and Race* (New York: Oxford University Press, January 2017; paperback, September 2018), Part VI, "Racisms and Neo-Racisms," 77–135; Naomi Zack, "Racism and Neo-Racisms," in *Philosophy of Race: An Introduction* (New York: Palgrave Macmillan, 2018), 149–74 (free download, https://link.springer.com/book/10.1007/978-3-319-78729-9).

5. Michael D. Shear and Maggie Haberman, "Trump's Temporary Halt to Immigration Is Part of Broader Plan, Stephen Miller Says," *New York Times*, April 24, 2020, updated July 23, 2020, https://www.nytimes.com/2020/04/24/us/politics/coronavirus-trump-immigration-stephen-miller.html.

6. Jack Kelly, "The Rich Are Riding Out the Coronavirus Pandemic Very Differently Than the Rest of Us," *Forbes*, April 1, 2020, https://www.forbes.com/sites/jackkelly/2020/04/01/the-rich-are-riding-out-the-coronavirus-pandemic-very-differently-than-the-rest-of-us/#16d3590dd34c.

7. Johnny Lopez, "Getting a Coronavirus Test Isn't Hard If You Are Rich and Famous," Radio.com, March 20, 2020, https://www.radio.com/news/getting-a-coronavirus-test-is-easy-for-the-rich-and-famous; David Mack, "What's the Point of a Coronavirus Test That Takes 19 Days for Results?" *BuzzFeed News*, July 25, 2020, https://www.buzzfeednews.com/article/davidmack/coronavirus-testing-delays-backlog.

8. See CIDRAP (Center for Infectious Disease Research and Policy), "Supply Chain Issues," July 24, 2020, https://www.cidrap.umn.edu/covid-19/supply-chain-issues.

9. For publications summarizing these findings, and debates about them, see the chapters in Naomi Zack, ed., *Oxford Handbook of Philosophy and Race* (New York: Oxford University Press, January 2017; paperback, September 2018), Part III, "Metaphysics and Philosophy of Science," 135–180. See also Naomi Zack, *Philosophy of Race: An Introduction* (New York: Palgrave Macmillan, Springer, 2018), chapter 3, "Race According to Biological Science," 47–70 (free download, https://link.springer.com/book/10.1007/978-3-319-78729-9).

10. See Claire Wang, "Trump's 'Kung Flu' Slur, Pervasive Scapegoating Recall a Brutal Decades-Old Hate Crime," NBC News, June 23, 2020; Elvia

Díaz, "COVID What? Gov. Doug Ducey Is Using Trump's 'Blame the Mexicans' Routine to Distract You," *Arizona Republic*, June 23, 2020, https://www.azcentral.com/story/opinion/op-ed/elviadiaz/2020/06/23/did-gov-doug-ducey-blame-mexicans-arizona-coronavirus-surge/3246567001/.

11. Bryan Armen Graham, "Tom Cotton Calls Slavery 'Necessary Evil' in Attack on *New York Times*' 1619 Project," *The Guardian*, July 26, 2020, https://www.theguardian.com/world/2020/jul/26/tom-cotton-slavery-necessary-evil-1619-project-new-york-times.

12. Tommy Beer, "New Poll Finds Americans Divided along Racial and Political Lines on the Issue of Reopening Schools," *Forbes*, July 23, 2020, https://www.forbes.com/sites/tommybeer/2020/07/23/new-poll-finds-americans-divided-along-racial-and-political-lines-on-the-issue-of-reopening-schools/#73fba1d74df4.

13. Jennifer Abbasi, "Taking a Closer Look at COVID-19, Health Inequities, and Racism," *JAMA Network*, published online June 29, 2020, https://jamanetwork.com/journals/jama/fullarticle/2767948.

14. Yancy, "COVID-19 and African Americans."

15. Kelly Glass, "Black Families Were Hit Hard by the Pandemic: The Effects on Children May Be Lasting," *New York Times*, July 29, 2020, https://www.nytimes.com/2020/06/29/parenting/coronavirus-black-children-inequality.html.

16. Jens Manuel Krogstad, Ana Gonzalez-Barrera, and Luis Noe-Bustamante, "U.S. Latinos among Hardest Hit by Pay Cuts, Job Losses Due to Coronavirus," Pew Research Center, April 3, 2020, https://www.pewresearch.org/fact-tank/2020/04/03/u-s-latinos-among-hardest-hit-by-pay-cuts-job-losses-due-to-coronavirus/.

17. Megan Mineiro, "DACA Ruling Safeguards Dreamers on the Front Lines of COVID-19," *Courthouse News Service*, June 18, 2020, https://www.courthousenews.com/daca-ruling-safeguards-dreamers-on-the-front-lines-of-covid-19/.

18. Helier Cheung, Zhaoyin Feng, and Boer Deng, "Coronavirus: What Attacks on Asians Reveal about American Identity," BBC News, May 27, 2020, https://www.bbc.com/news/world-us-canada-52714804.

19. Melany De La Cruz-Viesca, "Report Shows Major Effects of COVID-19 on Asian American Labor Force," Phys.org, July 23, 2020, https://phys.org/news/2020-07-major-effects-covid-asian-american.html.

20. Mark Magnier, "Asians in the US Least Likely to Get Coronavirus Infection Despite Racist Assumptions of Many, Data Suggests," SCMP.org, May 18, 2020, https://www.scmp.com/news/china/article/3084947/asians-us-least-likely-get-coronavirus-infection-data-suggests.

21. Liz Mineo, "For Native Americans, COVID-19 Is 'the Worst of Both Worlds at the Same Time,'" *Harvard Gazette*, May 8, 2020, https://news. harvard.edu/gazette/story/2020/05/the-impact-of-covid-19-on-native-american-communities/.

22. Kevin Abourezk, "Tribal Citizens Defend Coronavirus Checkpoints amid Threat from State," *Lakota Times*, May 13, 2020, https://www.lakota times.com/articles/tribal-citizens-defend-coronavirus-checkpoints-amid-threat-from-state/.

23. Arlie Hochschild and Anne Machung, *The Second Shift: Working Families and the Revolution at Home* (New York: Penguin Group, 1989/2003/2012).

24. Helen Lewis, "The Coronavirus Is a Disaster for Feminism: Pandemics Affect Men and Women Differently," *The Atlantic*, March 19, 2020, https://www.theatlantic.com/international/archive/2020/03/feminism-womens-rights-coronavirus-covid19/608302/.

25. Zaneta Thayer, "U.S. Coronavirus Advice Is Failing Pregnant Women," *Sapiens*, May 21, 2020, https://www.sapiens.org/body/covid-19-and-childbirth/.

26. See Shelley Wood, "COVID-19-Related Inflammatory Syndrome in Kids Needs Cardiac Follow-up," *tctMD*, June 10, 2020, https://www.tctmd. com/news/covid-19-related-inflammatory-syndrome-kids-needs-cardiac-follow; Jim Morrison, "What Scientists Know about How Children Spread COVID-19," smithsonianmag.com, July 23, 2020, https://www.smithsonian mag.com/science-nature/what-scientists-know-about-how-children-spread-covid-19-180975396/.

27. See Thomas Bahle, "Public Child Care in Europe: Historical Trajectories and New Directions," in K. Scheiwe and H. Willekens, eds., *Childcare and Preschool Development in Europe* (London: Palgrave Macmillan, 2009), 23–42.

28. See New York State Government, Childcare Services, Office of Family Services, https://ocfs.ny.gov/programs/childcare/.

29. Maclen Stanley, "Why the Increase in Domestic Violence during CO-VID-19? COVID-19 Has Triggered Common Factors Associated with Domestic Violence," *Psychology Today*, May 9, 2020, https://www.psychologytoday. com/us/blog/making-sense-chaos/202005/why-the-increase-in-domestic-violence-during-covid-19.

30. See National Council on Aging (NCOA), "COVID-19 Resources for Older Adults & Caregivers," https://www.ncoa.org/ncoa_acf/covid-19-resources-for-older-adults/.

31. R. Stepler, American Psychological Association, "By the Numbers: Older Adults Living Alone," *Monitor on Psychology* 47, no. 5 (2016): 9 (print version), https://www.apa.org/monitor/2016/05/numbers.

32. Chris Lee, "8 in 10 People Who Have Died of COVID-19 Were Age 65 or Older—But the Share Varies by State," KFF (Kaiser Family Foundation),

July 24, 2020, https://www.kff.org/coronavirus-covid-19/press-release/8-in-10-people-who-have-died-of-covid-19-were-age-65-or-older-but-the-share-varies-by-state/.

33. Robert Roy Britt, "Here's Who's Dying from COVID-19 in the United States: Data and New Research Reveal All Age Groups Are at Risk, from Children to Middle Age and Beyond," *Elemental*, Medium, May 11, 2020, https://elemental.medium.com/its-not-just-sick-old-people-who-die-from-covid-19-bc9251989bc8.

34. Jonathan Chait, "Trump Brags That He Repeated 5 Words in a Row on 'Difficult' Dementia Test," *Intelligencer, New York Magazine*, July 22, 2020, https://nymag.com/intelligencer/2020/07/trump-repeated-5-words-person-woman-man-camera-tx-dementia-cognitive-test.html.

35. Michael E. Newman, "COVID-19 Story Tip: Herd Immunity Is a Dangerous Strategy for Fighting COVID-19, Says Johns Hopkins Expert," Medical Xpress, Johns Hopkins University, August 26, 2020, https://medicalxpress.com/news/2020-08-herd-immunity-dangerous-strategy-covid-.html; Sheryl Gay Stolberg, "White House Embraces a Declaration from Scientists That Opposes Lockdowns and Relies on 'Herd Immunity,'" *New York Times*, October 13, 2020, https://www.nytimes.com/2020/10/13/world/white-house-embraces-a-declaration-from-scientists-that-opposes-lockdowns-and-relies-on-herd-immunity.html.

36. CDC, "People with Disabilities," April 7, 2020, https://www.cdc.gov/coronavirus/2019-ncov/need-extra-precautions/people-with-disabilities.html.

37. Center for Disability Studies, "'We're Being Punished Again': How People with Intellectual Disabilities Are Experiencing the Pandemic," originally published April 6, 2020, by Vox, https://www.cds.udel.edu/item/were-being-punished-again-how-people-with-intellectual-disabilities-are-experiencing-the-pandemic/.

38. Reform Austin Staff, "One Texas County Is Turning COVID-19 Patients Away to Die," *Reform Austin*, July 22, 2020, https://www.reformaustin.org/coronavirus/one-texas-county-is-turning-covid-19-patients-away-to-die/.

39. Brendan Saloner, Kalind Parish, Julie A. Ward, et al., "COVID-19 Cases and Deaths in Federal and State Prisons," *JAMA Network*, July 8, 2020, https://jamanetwork.com/journals/jama/fullarticle/2768249.

40. Holly Honderich and Shrai Popat, "Coronavirus: Can This California Prison Save Itself from Covid-19?" BBC News, July 27, 2020, https://www.bbc.com/news/world-us-canada-53476208.

41. See endnote 3, supra.

42. Shan Li and Ben Chapman, "New York City Subway Begins Nightly Shutdowns for Coronavirus Cleaning," *Wall Street Journal*, updated May 6,

2020, https://www.wsj.com/articles/new-york-city-subway-begins-nightly-shutdowns-for-coronavirus-cleaning-11588767945.

43. Courtney Gross, "Close to 20 Percent of NYC Hotels Are Housing the Homeless," Spectrum News1, NYC, June 25, 2020, https://www.ny1.com/nyc/all-boroughs/homelessness/2020/06/25/close-to-20-percent-of-nyc-hotels-are-housing-the-homeless.

44. CDC, "Assessment of SARS-CoV-2 Infection Prevalence in Homeless Shelters: Four U.S. Cities, March 27–April 15, 2020," *Morbidity and Mortality Weekly Report* 69, no. 17 (May 1, 2020): 521–22, https://www.cdc.gov/mmwr/volumes/69/wr/mm6917e1.htm.

45. Kristine Liao, "California's Homeless Population Faces Wildfire Smoke and COVID-19," *Global Citizen*, September 11, 2020, https://www.global citizen.org/en/content/california-homeless-face-wildfire-smoke-covid-19/.

46. Médecins Sans Frontières, "Facts and Figures about the Coronavirus Disease Outbreak: COVID-19, What We Know about This Pandemic and How MSF Teams Are Responding," https://www.doctorswithoutborders.org/covid19; idem, USA, https://www.doctorswithoutborders.org/what-we-do/news-stories/news/msf-helps-respond-needs-vulnerable-communities-us-during-covid-19.

47. For discussion of the general problem with homelessness in the United States and further sources, see Naomi Zack, *Reviving the Social Compact: Inclusive Citizenship in an Age of Extreme Politics* (Lanham, MD: Rowman & Littlefield, 2018), chapter 8, "Homelessness and Monetization," 131–46.

48. Liao, "California's Homeless Population Faces Wildfire Smoke and COVID-19."

49. See Daniel Burke, "Coronavirus Preys on What Terrifies Us: Dying Alone," CNN News, March 29, 2020, https://www.cnn.com/2020/03/29/world/funerals-dying-alone-coronavirus/index.html; Robin Wright, "How Loneliness from Coronavirus Isolation Takes Its Own Toll," *New Yorker Magazine*, March 23, 2020, https://www.newyorker.com/news/our-columnists/how-loneliness-from-coronavirus-isolation-takes-its-own-toll.

50. For fact checks for this subsection, see Burke, "Coronavirus Preys on What Terrifies Us: Dying Alone," and Wright, "How Loneliness from Coronavirus Isolation Takes Its Own Toll."

5. POLICE REFORM

1. Judith A. Beeman, editor in chief, *United States Attorneys' Bulletin* (US Department of Justice) 39, no. 7 (July 15, 1991): 30.

2. Krista Aniston, "Al Sharpton," Top 983 Police Quotes, *Quotes Study*, October 20, 2020, https://quotesstudy.com/about-police-quotes/.

3. Ta-Nehisi Coates, *Between the World and Me* (New York: Random House, 2015), 78.

4. Jeremy W. Peters, "Asked about Black Americans Killed by Police, Trump Says, 'So Are White People,'" *New York Times*, July 14, 2020, https://www.nytimes.com/2020/07/14/us/politics/trump-white-people-killed-by-police.html.

5. CNN, "Biden: The Original Sin of Slavery Stains Our Country Today," *Microsoft News*, May 29, 2020, https://www.msn.com/en-us/news/politics/biden-the-original-sin-of-slavery-stains-our-country-today/vp-BB14M9S7.

6. Ian Schwartz, "Trump Ad on What Happens If Police Are Defunded: 'Our Estimated Wait Time Is Currently 5 Days,'" *Real Clear Politics*, July 2, 2020, https://www.realclearpolitics.com/video/2020/07/02/trump_ad_on_what_happens_if_police_are_defunded_our_estimated_wait_time_is_currently_5_days.html.

7. For US police structure organization, see "Types of Law Enforcement Agencies," Discover Policing, https://www.discoverpolicing.org/explore-the-field/types-of-law-enforcement-agencies/; Department of Homeland Security, "Operational and Support Components," https://www.dhs.gov/operational-and-support-components; Wikipedia, "Law Enforcement in the United States," https://en.wikipedia.org/wiki/Law_enforcement_in_the_United_States; *JRank Law Library*, "Police: Organization and Management, the American System of Policing," https://law.jrank.org/pages/1668/Police-Organization-Management-American-system-policing.html; *National Law Enforcement Officers Memorial Fund*, "Law Enforcement Facts," https://nleomf.org/facts-figures/law-enforcement-facts.

8. Drew DeSilver, Michael Lipka, and Dalia Fahmy, "10 Things We Know about Race and Policing in the U.S.," Pew Research Center, June 3, 2020, https://www.pewresearch.org/fact-tank/2020/06/03/10-things-we-know-about-race-and-policing-in-the-u-s/.

9. Barbara Armacost, "The Organizational Reasons Police Departments Don't Change," *Harvard Business Review*, August 19, 2016, https://hbr.org/2016/08/the-organizational-reasons-police-departments-dont-change.

10. Anthony Fisher, "Why It's So Hard to Stop Bad Cops from Getting New Police Jobs," *Reason*, September 20, 2016, https://reason.com/2016/09/30/why-its-so-hard-to-stop-bad-cops-from-ge/.

11. Noam Scheiber, Farah Stockman, and J. David Goodman, "How Police Unions Became Such Powerful Opponents to Reform Efforts," *New York Times*, June 6, 2020, updated June 20, 2020, https://www.nytimes.com/2020/06/06/us/police-unions-minneapolis-kroll.html.

12. Parts of this section—especially the discussion of US Supreme Court cases—rely on parts of Naomi Zack, *White Privilege and Black Rights: The Injustice of U.S. Police Racial Profiling and Homicide* (Lanham, MD: Rowman & Littlefield, 2015), chapter 3, 63–92.

13. Michelle Alexander, *The New Jim Crow: Mass Incarceration in the Age of Colorblindness* (New York: The New Press, Kindle Edition, 2012), 200. Cited by Janine Jones in "Can We Imagine *This* Happening to a White Boy?" in George Yancy and Janine Jones, eds., *Pursuing Trayvon Martin: Historical Contexts and Contemporary Manifestations of Racial Dynamics* (Lanham, MD: Lexington Books, 2013), 142.

14. Melissa Segura, "On the Day George Floyd Died, Police across the US Shot and Killed at Least Five Other Men," *BuzzFeed News*, June 27, 2020, https://www.buzzfeednews.com/article/melissasegura/george-floyd-other-men-killed-by-police.

15. Lawrence Kobilinsky, forensics expert and chair of the Department of Sciences at the John Jay College of Criminal Justice in New York City, commenting on death of Tamir Rice. Kobilinsky is here making the point that homicide has two meanings in law: death of one human being by another, and criminal death of one human being by another. See "Homicide Definition," *FindLaw*, http://criminal.findlaw.com/criminal-charges/homicide-definition.html; *Crimesider* Staff, "Autopsy Calls Tamir Rice Shooting Death a Homicide," CBS News /AP, December 12, 2014, http://www.cbsnews.com/news/medical-examiner-rules-tamir-rices-death-a-homicide/.

16. Martin Kaste, "It's a Complicated Relationship between Prosecutors, Police," *All Things Considered*, NPR, December 4, 2020, https://www.npr.org/2014/12/04/368529402/its-a-complicated-relationship-between-prosecutors-police.

17. *Graham v. Connor*, 490 U.S. 389 (1989).

18. *Plumhoff et al. v. Rickard*, US Supreme Court, October Term, 2013, http://www.supremecourt.gov/opinions/13pdf/12-1117_1bn5.pdf.

19. James C. McKinley Jr. and Al Baker, "Grand Jury System, with Exceptions, Favors the Police in Fatalities," *New York Times*, December 7, 2014, https://www.nytimes.com/2014/12/08/nyregion/grand-juries-seldom-charge-police-officers-in-fatal-actions.html?. (McKinley and Baker derive their figures from research by Philip M. Stinson, criminologist at Bowling Green State University, http://works.bepress.com/philip_stinson/.)

20. Wikipedia, "Lists of Killings by Law Enforcement Officers in the United States," July 13, 2020, https://en.wikipedia.org/wiki/Lists_of_killings_by_law_enforcement_officers_in_the_United_States.

21. Ibid., 396–97.

22. See Mary Reichard, "Lethal Force in Ferguson and Beyond," December 1, 2014, *World*, Real Matters/WNG.org, https://world.wng.org/2014/12/lethal_force_in_ferguson_and_beyond.

23. For an update on the application of qualified immunity, see Andrew Chung, Lawrence Hurley, Jackie Botts, Januta Andrea, and Guillermo Gomez, "Excessive Force, Zero Justice, for Cops Who Kill," Reuters, May 8, 2020, https://www.reuters.com/investigates/special-report/usa-police-immunity-scotus/.

24. *Tennessee v. Garner*, 471 U.S. 1 (1985), FindLaw, 7–12, http://caselaw.lp.findlaw.com/scripts/getcase.pl?court=US&vol=471&invol=1.

25. *Terry v. Ohio*. 392 I/S/ 1 (1968), no. 67, http://scholar.google.com/scholar_case?case=17773604035873288886&q=terry+v.+ohio,+us+supreme+court&hl=en&as_sdt=3,38.

26. Quotations from *Terry v. Ohio*, 16–27.

27. James Hill, "Milwaukee Police Officer Not Charged in Fatal Shooting," December 22, 2014, ABC News, http://abcnews.go.com/US/milwaukee-police-officer-charged-fatal-shooting/story?id=27767944.

28. See Paula Ioanide, *The Emotional Politics of Racism: How Feelings Trump Facts in an Era of Colorblindness* (Stanford, CA: Stanford University Press, 2015); R. Caldara and L. Vizioli, "The Speed of Race" [Abstract], *Journal of Vision* 10, no. 7 (2010): 699, 699a, http://www.journalofvision.org/content/10/7/699, DOI:10.1167/10.7.699.

29. E. Bittner, "Quasi-Military Organization of Police," in *Police and Society: Touchstone Readings*, Victor E. Kappeler, ed., National Criminal Justice Reference Service (NCJRS), NCJ-151401 (1995): 173–84, https://www.ncjrs.gov/App/Publications/abstract.aspx?ID=151410.

30. Sarah Lawrence and Bobby McCarthy, "What Works in Community Policing," Chief Justice Earl Warren Institute on Law and Social Policy University of California, Berkeley School of Law, November 2013, https://www.law.berkeley.edu/files/What_Works_in_Community_Policing.pdf.

31. Richard E. Adams, William M. Rohe, Thomas A. Arcury, "Implementing Community-Oriented Policing: Organizational Change and Street Officer Attitudes," *Crime and Delinquency*, July 1, 2002, https://doi.org/10.1177/0011128702048003003.

32. Jerry Abramson, "10 Cities Making Real Progress Since the Launch of the 21st Century Policing Task Force," White House/President Barack Obama, May 18, 2015, https://obamawhitehouse.archives.gov/blog/2015/05/18/10-cities-making-real-progress-launch-21st-century-policing-task-force.

33. Gabriel T. Rubin, "Protests Draw Attention to Trump-Requested Cuts to Community Policing and Mediation Programs at the Justice Department," *Wall Street Journal*, June 5, 2020, https://www.wsj.com/articles/democrats-

push-to-block-trump-requested-cuts-to-community-policing-programs-11591349402.

34. Donald J. Trump, "Executive Order on Safe Policing for Safe Communities," June 16, 2020, https://www.whitehouse.gov/presidential-actions/executive-order-safe-policing-safe-communities/.

35. Brenda Breslauer, Kit Ramgopal, Kenzi Abou-Sabe, and Stephanie Gosk, "Camden, N.J., Disbanded Its Police Force: Here's What Happened Next," NBC News, June 22, 2020, https://www.nbcnews.com/news/us-news/new-jersey-city-disbanded-its-police-force-here-s-what-n1231677; see also this Twitter photo of Camden during the George Floyd protests, https://twitter.com/CamdenCountyPD/status/1266882383980216320?s=19.

36. Naomi Zack, *White Privilege and Black Rights: The Injustice of U.S. Police Racial Profiling and Homicide* (Lanham, MD: Rowman & Littlefield, 2015), 100.

37. Jamein Cunningham and Rob Gillezeau, "Don't Shoot! The Impact of Historical African American Protest on Police Killings of Civilians," *Journal of Quantitative Criminology* (2019): 1–34, 10.1007/s10940-019-09443-8.

6. EDUCATION

1. Benjamin Franklin, "Proposals Relating to the Education of Youth in Pensilvania [sic], 1747," National Humanities Center Resource Toolbox, Becoming American: The British Atlantic Colonies, 1690–1763, http://nationalhumanitiescenter.org/pds/becomingamer/ideas/text4/franklinproposals.pdf.

2. Samuel Rodenhizer, "Change Is the End Result of All True Learning," *Quotation Celebration*, August 27, 2018, https://quotationcelebration.wordpress.com/2018/08/27/change-is-the-end-result-of-all-true-learning-leo-buscaglia/.

3. Friedrich Nietzsche, "Reason in Philosophy," Sec. 1, *Twilight of the Idols: Or How to Philosophize with the Hammer*, trans. Richard Polt (Indianapolis, IN: Hackett, 1997/2009), 18, http://www.faculty.umb.edu/gary_zabel/Phil_100/Nietzsche_files/Friedrich-Nietzsche-Twilight-of-the-Idols-or-How-to-Philosophize-With-the-Hammer-Translated-by-Richard-Polt.pdf.

4. For these facts and numbers, see National Center for Education Statistics, "Back to School Statistics," Educational Institutions, Expenditures, Fast Facts, https://nces.ed.gov/fastfacts/display.asp?id=372#PK12_enrollment and https://nces.ed.gov/fastfacts/display.asp?id=84, consulted August 18, 2020; Organisation for Economic Co-operation and Development (OECD), "Education at a Glance," 2012, https://www.oecd.org/unitedstates/CN%20-%20United

%20States.pdf; Wikipedia, "Education in the United States," https://en.m.
wikipedia.org/wiki/Education_in_the_United_States.

5. N. S. Wigginton, R. M. Cunningham, R. H. Katz, M. E. Lidstrom, K. A.
Moler, D. Wirtz, and M. T. Zuber, "Moving Academic Research Forward
during COVID-19," *Science* 368, issue 6496 (June 12, 2020): 1190–92, DOI:
10.1126/science.abc5599, https://science.sciencemag.org/content/368/6496/
1190.long.

6. Jessica Bursztynsky, "Apple Becomes First U.S. Company to Reach a $2
Trillion Market Cap," CNBC, August 19, 2020, https://www.cnbc.com/2020/
08/19/apple-reaches-2-trillion-market-cap.html.

7. For GNP and US population, see *Trading Economics*, https://trading
economics.com/united-states/gross-national-product; Google, https://www.
google.com/search?client=firefox-b-1-d&q=us+population.

8. "The Coronavirus Spring: The Historic Closing of U.S. Schools, July 1,
2020," *Education Week*, https://www.edweek.org/ew/section/multimedia/the-
coronavirus-spring-the-historic-closing-of.html.

9. Ibid.

10. "Pediatricians, Educators and Superintendents Urge a Safe Return to
School This Fall" (news release), July 10, 2020, https://services.aap.org/en/
news-room/news-releases/aap/2020/pediatricians-educators-and-
superintendents-urge-a-safe-return-to-school-this-fall/.

11. R. T. Leeb, S. Price, S. Sliwa, et al., "COVID-19 Trends among School-
Aged Children: United States, March 1–September 19, 2020," *Morbidity and
Mortality Weekly Report* (CDC) 69 (2020): 1410–15, DOI: http://dx.doi.org/
10.15585/mmwr.mm6939e2, https://www.cdc.gov/mmwr/volumes/69/wr/
mm6939e2.htm#suggestedcitation.

12. American College Health Association, ACHA Guidelines, "Considera-
tions for Reopening Institutions of Higher Education in the COVID-19 Era,"
May 7, 2020, https://www.acha.org/documents/resources/guidelines/ACHA_
Considerations_for_Reopening_IHEs_in_the_COVID-19_Era_May2020.pdf.

13. See Kai Kupferschmidt, "'A Completely New Culture of Doing Research': Coronavirus Outbreak Changes How Scientists Communicate," *Science*, February 26, 2020, https://www.sciencemag.org/news/2020/02/
completely-new-culture-doing-research-coronavirus-outbreak-changes-how-
scientists; P. R. Padala, A. M. Jendro, and K. P. Padala, "Conducting Clinical
Research during the COVID-19 Pandemic: Investigator and Participant Perspectives," *JMIR Public Health and Surveillance* 6, no. 2 (2020): e18887, published April 6, 2020, DOI:10.2196/18887, https://www.ncbi.nlm.nih.gov/pmc/
articles/PMC7141248/.

14. N. S. Wigginton et al., "Moving Academic Research Forward during COVID-19," *Science* 368, no. 6496 (June 12, 2020).

15. *College Tuition Compare*, "Ivy League 2020 Tuition Comparison and 2021 Estimation," http://blog.collegetuitioncompare.com/2015/05/ivy-league-2015-2016-estimated-tuition.html?m=1.

16. Zack Friedman, "Hollywood Celebrities Charged in Major College Admissions Scandal," Personal Finance, *Forbes*, March 12, 2020, https://www.forbes.com/sites/zackfriedman/2019/03/12/hollywood-celebrities-charged-in-major-college-admissions-scandal/#d30b53f1dc54.

17. Rebecca Zwick, "Assessment in American Higher Education: The Role of Admissions Tests," *Annals of the American Academy of Political and Social Sciences*, May 16, 2019, https://journals.sagepub.com/doi/abs/10.1177/0002716219843469, https://doi.org/10.1177/0002716219843469.

18. Eliza Shapiro and K. K. Rebecca Lai, "How New York's Elite Public Schools Lost Their Black and Hispanic Students," *New York Times*, June 3, 2019, https://www.nytimes.com/interactive/2019/06/03/nyregion/nyc-public-schools-black-hispanic-students.html.

19. Richard Breen, "Education and Intergenerational Social Mobility in the US and Four European Countries," *Oxford Review of Economic Policy* 35, issue 3 (Autumn 2019): 445–66, https://doi.org/10.1093/oxrep/grz013.

20. Dana Goldstein, "'Big Mess' Looms If Schools Don't Get Billions to Reopen Safely," *New York Times*, July 29, 2020, https://www.nytimes.com/2020/07/09/us/schools-reopening-trump.html; Hardy Murphy, "Making Schools Safe Will Take More Than Wiping Down Surfaces," *The Conversation*, July 31, 2020, https://theconversation.com/poor-minority-students-at-dilapidated-schools-face-added-risks-amid-talk-of-reopening-classrooms-142892.

21. USDA, "Find Meals for Kids When Schools Are Closed," US Department of Agriculture, Food and Nutrition Service, https://www.fns.usda.gov/meals4kids.

22. Emily Bazelon, "Will This Be a Lost Year for America's School Children?" Education Issue, *New York Times*, September 11, 2020, https://www.nytimes.com/interactive/2020/09/11/magazine/covid-school-reopenings.html.

23. George Psacharopoulos, Harry Patrinos, Victoria Collis, and Emiliana Vegas, "The COVID-19 Cost of School Closures," *Brookings*, April 29, 2020, https://www.brookings.edu/blog/education-plus-development/2020/04/29/the-covid-19-cost-of-school-closures/.

24. Douglas B. Holt, "Does Cultural Capital Structure American Consumption?" *Journal of Consumer Research* 25, issue 1 (June 1998): 1–25, https://doi.org/10.1086/209523.

25. Philippe Ariès, *Centuries of Childhood*, trans. Robert Baldick (New York: Alfred A. Knopf, 1962), 92–93, 99.

26. Michael T. Nietzel, "Five Reasons 2020 Will Be the Year of the Student Protest," *Forbes,* July 10, 2020, https://www.forbes.com/sites/michaeltnietzel/2020/07/10/five-reasons-2020-is-the-year-of-the-student-protest/#65d8ddd73ce7.

27. David L. Hildebrand, *Dewey: A Beginner's Guide* (Oxford, UK: One World Books, 2008), 128 (from John Dewey "Between Two Worlds," 1944, LW17: 463), https://epdf.pub/queue/dewey-a-beginners-guide-beginners-guide-oneworld.html.

28. John Dewey, *Moral Principles in Education*, II: The Moral Training Given by the School Community (Chicago, IL: Houghton Mifflin, 1909) (1897a, EW5: 61–62), http://catalog.lambertvillelibrary.org/texts/American/dewey/moral/moral.htm.

29. Matt Richtel, "Looking to Reopen, Colleges Become Labs for Coronavirus Tests and Tracking Apps," *New York Times*, August 30, 2020, https://www.nytimes.com/2020/08/30/us/colleges-coronavirus-research.html.

30. James D. Walsh, "The Coming Disruption: Scott Galloway Predicts a Handful of Elite Cyborg Universities Will Soon Monopolize Higher Education," Intelligencer, *New York Magazine*, May 2020, https://nymag.com/intelligencer/2020/05/scott-galloway-future-of-college.html. See also "The Professor G. Show with Scott Galloway," *Westwood One Podcasts*, http://www.westwoodonepodcasts.com/pods/the-prof-g-show-with-scott-galloway/.

31. Shawn Hubler, "Colleges Slash Budgets in the Pandemic, with 'Nothing Off-Limits,'" *New York Times*, October 28, 2020, https://www.nytimes.com/2020/10/26/us/colleges-coronavirus-budget-cuts.html.

32. K. R. Myers, W. Y. Tham, Y. Yin, et al., "Unequal Effects of the COVID-19 Pandemic on Scientists," *Nature Human Behaviour*, July 15, 2020, https://doi.org/10.1038/s41562-020-0921-y, https://www.nature.com/articles/s41562-020-0921-y.

33. Emily Peck, "COVID-19 Is a Rolling Disaster for Working Mothers," *Knowledia*, August 19, 2020, https://news.knowledia.com/CA/en/articles/covid-19-is-a-rolling-disaster-for-working-mothers-96ab3c053c37ff6dab061a3fc14faccba8c0a489.

34. Porsche Moran, "Lifestyle Advice," Investopedia, March 21, 2020, https://www.investopedia.com/financial-edge/0112/how-much-is-a-homemaker-worth.aspx.

35. Naomi Zack, "Suffrage Comes with Obligations. Voting Is Only the First," *Forward*, August 18, 2020, https://forward.com/culture/452827/suffrage-obligations-voting-only-the-first-19th-amendment-centennial/.

36. National Center for Education Statistics, "Enrollment," Fast Facts, https://nces.ed.gov/fastfacts/display.asp?id=98.

7. ECONOMY

1. "Ned Beatty: Arthur Jensen," *Network*, Metro-Goldwyn-Mayer (1976), IMDB.com, https://www.imdb.com/title/tt0074958/characters/nm0000885.

2. John Locke, "Some Considerations of the Consequences of the Lowering of Interest and Rising the Value of Money," in Patrick Hyde Kelly, ed., *Locke on Money*, vol. 1 (Oxford: Oxford Clarendon Press, 1991), 233–34. See also Naomi Zack, "Lockean Money, Globalism and Indigenism," in Catherine Wilson, ed., "Civilization and Oppression," *Canadian Journal of Philosophy* 25 (1999): 31–53.

3. Siblis Research, "Total Market Value of U.S. Stock Market," June 30, 2020, https://siblisresearch.com/data/us-stock-market-value/.

4. Wikipedia, "CARES Act," August 16, 2020, https://en.wikipedia.org/wiki/CARES_Act.

5. See Zack, "Lockean Money, Globalism and Indigenism."

6. Robert Hockett and Aaron James, *Money from Nothing: Or, Why We Should Stop Worrying about Debt and Learn to Love the Federal Reserve* (Brooklyn, NY/London: Melville House, 2020).

7. Jim Chappelow, "Gross National Income (GNI)," Investopedia, August 20, 2020, https://www.investopedia.com/terms/g/gross-national-income-gni.asp.

8. Peter Carleton, "What Is the Gross National Product (GNP)?" *Investing Answers*, August 22, 2020, https://investinganswers.com/dictionary/g/gross-national-product-gnp.

9. Jim Chappelow, "Gross National Income (GNI)," Investopedia, April 6, 2020, https://www.investopedia.com/terms/g/gross-national-income-gni.asp.

10. *IndexMundi*, Home, "United States GDP: Composition by Sector," https://www.indexmundi.com/united_states/gdp_composition_by_sector.html.

11. Investopedia, "Sectors," https://www.investopedia.com/terms/s/sector-breakdown.asp.

12. Bureau of Economic Analysis (BEA), "US Economy at a Glance," July 30, 2020, https://www.bea.gov/news/glance.

13. Bureau of Economic Analysis (BEA), "US Economy at a Glance," October 29, 2020, https://www.bea.gov/news/2020/gross-domestic-product-third-quarter-2020-advance-estimate.

14. James B. Stewart and Alan Rappeport, "Steven Mnuchin Tried to Save the Economy. Not Even His Family Is Happy," *New York Times*, August 30,

2020, https://www.nytimes.com/2020/08/30/business/steven-mnuchin-trump-economy.html.

15. US Department of Labor, "The Employment Situation—August 2020," News Release, Bureau of Labor Statistics, September 4, 2020, https://www.bls.gov/news.release/pdf/empsit.pdf.

16. US Bureau of Labor Statistics, "Economy at a Glance," October 28, 2020, https://www.bls.gov/eag/eag.us.htm.

17. Investopedia, "Price-to-Earnings Ratio—P/E Ratio," https://www.investopedia.com/terms/p/price-earningsratio.asp.

18. Al Root, "Next Year Looks Rocky for the Stock Market No Matter Who Wins the Election," *Barron's*, updated September 14, 2020, https://www.barrons.com/articles/it-doesnt-matter-if-its-trump-or-bidennext-year-looks-rocky-for-the-stock-market-51599868976.

19. Randall W. Forsyth, "Up and Down Wall Street: One More for 2020," *Barron's*, October 5, 2020, 9–10.

20. CDC, "Scientific Brief: Community Use of Cloth Masks to Control the Spread of SARS-CoV-2," November 10, 2020, https://www.cdc.gov/coronavirus/2019-ncov/more/masking-science-sars-cov2.html; *Healthline*, "Here's Exactly Where We Are with Vaccines and Treatments for COVID-19," November 9, 2020, https://www.healthline.com/health-news/heres-exactly-where-were-at-with-vaccines-and-treatments-for-covid-19.

21. National Conference of State Legislatures, "COVID-19: Essential Workers in the States," https://www.ncsl.org/research/labor-and-employment/covid-19-essential-workers-in-the-states.aspx.

22. Celine McNicholas and Margaret Poydock, "Who Are Essential Workers? A Comprehensive Look at Their Wages, Demographics, and Unionization Rates," *Economic Policy Institute*, May 19, 2020, https://www.epi.org/blog/who-are-essential-workers-a-comprehensive-look-at-their-wages-demographics-and-unionization-rates/.

23. Megan Molteni, "Why Meatpacking Plants Have Become Covid-19 Hot Spots," *WIRED*, May 7, 2020, https://www.wired.com/story/why-meatpacking-plants-have-become-covid-19-hot-spots/.

24. John Mirowsky and Catherine E. Ross, *Education, Social Status, and Health* (New York: Routledge, 2003).

25. Francine D. Blau, Josefine Koebe, and Pamela A. Meyerhofer, "Essential and Frontline Workers in the COVID-19 Crisis," *Econofact*, April 30, 2020, https://econofact.org/essential-and-frontline-workers-in-the-covid-19-crisis.

26. Teresa Ghilarducci, "Why Essential Workers Deserve COVID-19 Hazard Pay," *Forbes*, June 28, 2020, https://www.forbes.com/sites/teresaghilarducci/2020/06/28/essential-workers-need-hazard-pay--hike-pay-by-2900-per-month/#3e5a87a91ce3.

27. Jeanna Smialek, Ben Casselman, and Gillian Friedman, "Workers Face Permanent Job Losses as the Virus Persists," *New York Times*, October 3, 2020, https://www.nytimes.com/2020/10/03/business/economy/coronavirus-permanent-job-losses.html.

28. John Authers, "When Plagues Pass, Labor Gets the Upper Hand: For Centuries, Pandemics Have Been Followed by Slower Growth and Social Unrest," *Bloomberg Opinion*, April 5, 2020, https://www.bloomberg.com/opinion/articles/2020-04-05/when-plagues-pass-labor-gets-the-upper-hand.

29. Mimi Abramovitz, "Economic Crises, Neoliberalism, and the US Welfare State: Trends, Outcomes and Political Struggle," in Carolyn Noble, Helle Strauss, and Brian Littlechild, eds., *Global Social Work: Crossing Borders, Blurring Boundaries* (Australia: Sydney University Press, 2014), 225–40, accessed August 26, 2020, http://www.jstor.org/stable/j.ctv1fxm2q.20.

30. Sabri Ben-Achour, Candace Manriquez Wrenn, Erika Soderstrom, and Alex Schroeder, "The RNC and DNC Painted Very Different Pictures of the U.S. Economy," *Marketplace*, August 28, 2020, https://www.marketplace.org/2020/08/28/rnc-trump-dnc-biden-economy-pandemic/.

31. Naomi Klein, *The Shock Doctrine: The Rise of Disaster Capitalism* (New York: Henry Holt, 2008).

32. Amber Colón Núñez, "The Coronvirus Crisis Is Capitalism in Action: Here's How the Left Can Respond," *In These Times*, March 27, 2020, https://inthesetimes.com/article/coronavirus-crisis-disaster-capitalism-naomi-klein-covid-19.

33. Keeanga-Yamahtta Taylor, "How Do We Change America: The Quest to Transform This Country Cannot Be Limited to Challenging Its Brutal Police," *New Yorker*, June 8, 2020, https://www.newyorker.com/news/our-columnists/how-do-we-change-america.

34. Blackpast, "(1951) We Charge Genocide," July 15, 2011, https://www.blackpast.org/global-african-history/primary-documents-global-african-history/we-charge-genocide-historic-petition-united-nations-relief-crime-united-states-government-against/.

35. Federal Safety Net, "US Poverty Statistics," September 19, 2020, http://federalsafetynet.com/us-poverty-statistics.html.

36. Thomas Piketty, *Capital in the Twenty-First Century*, trans. Arthur Goldhammer (Cambridge, MA: Harvard University Press, 2014).

37. Slavoj Žižek, *Pandemic! COVID-19 Shakes the World* (New York: OR Books, LLC/Polity Press, 2020), 95–107.

38. See Naomi Zack, *Progressive Anonymity: From Identity Politics to Evidence-Based Government* (Lanham, MD: Rowman & Littlefield, 2020), chapter 5, "Evidence-Based Government and Its Obstacles," 87–108.

39. Souheil El-Masri and Graham Tipple, "Natural Disaster, Mitigation and Sustainability: The Case of Developing Countries," *International Planning Studies* 7, issue 2 (2002): 157–75, DOI:10.1080/13563470220132236.

40. N. Ahmed, S. Thompson, and M. Glaser, "Global Aquaculture Productivity, Environmental Sustainability, and Climate Change Adaptability," *Environmental Management* 63 (2019): 159–72, https://doi.org/10.1007/s00267-018-1117-3.

8. MEDIA

1. Emily S. Rueb and Derrick Bryson Taylor, "Obama on Call-Out Culture: 'That's Not Activism,'" *New York Times*, October 31, 2019, https://www.nytimes.com/2019/10/31/us/politics/obama-woke-cancel-culture.html.

2. *The Godfather: Part II*, "Keep your friends close, but your enemies closer," https://www.youtube.com/watch?v=DfHJDLoGInM.

3. Editors of the *Encyclopedia Britannica*, "The *New York Times*," https://www.britannica.com/topic/The-New-York-Times.

4. Cotton's op-ed and responses to it can be found at Tom Cotton, "Opinion: Send in the Troops," *New York Times*, June 3, 4, 5, 2020, https://www.nytimes.com/2020/06/03/opinion/tom-cotton-protests-military.html.

5. Marc Tracy, "James Bennet Resigns as *New York Times* Opinion Editor," *New York Times*, July 7, 2020, https://www.nytimes.com/2020/06/07/business/media/james-bennet-resigns-nytimes-op-ed.html.

6. See Lara Ehrlich, "President Trump Claims the Media Peddles Fake News: Has It Made Itself an Easy Target?" *Com/Talk*, College of Communication, Boston University, June 12, 2020, https://www.bu.edu/com/comtalk/the-war-on-fake-news/.

7. Robert D. Leigh, ed., *A Free and Responsible Press: A General Report on Mass Communication: Newspapers, Motion Pictures, Radio, Magazines, and Books, by the Commission on Freedom of the Press* (Chicago and London: University of Chicago Press, 1947/Midway Press, 1974).

8. Michael Luo, "How Can the Press Best Serve a Democratic Society?" *New Yorker*, July 11, 2020, https://www.newyorker.com/news/the-future-of-democracy/how-can-the-press-best-serve-democracy.

9. John Stuart Mill, *On Liberty*, Excerpts, *Open Mind*, 22, http://openmindplatform.org/wp-content/uploads/2018/02/John-Stuart-Mill_On-Liberty_Excerpts.pdf.

10. Colleen Walsh, "Must We Allow Symbols of Racism on Public Land?" National & World Affairs, *Harvard Gazette*, June 19, 2020, https://news.

harvard.edu/gazette/story/2020/06/historian-puts-the-push-to-remove-confederate-statues-in-context/.

11. See Charles B. Dew, *Apostles of Disunion: Southern Secession Commissioners and the Causes of the Civil War* (Charlottesville: University of Virginia Press, 2001/2017).

12. Travis Timmerman, "A Case for Removing Confederate Monuments," in Bob Fischer, ed., *Ethics, Left and Right: The Moral Issues That Divide Us* (New York: Oxford University Press, 2020), 513–22, and https://philpapers.org/archive/TIMACF.pdf.

13. Rachel Scully and James Bikales, "A List of the Statues across the US Toppled, Vandalized or Officially Removed amid Protests," *The Hill*, June 12, 2020, https://thehill.com/homenews/state-watch/502492-list-statues-toppled-vandalized-removed-protests.

14. Rodney A. Young, "Great Emancipator, Supplicant Slave: The Freedman's Memorial to Abraham Lincoln," *Slaves, Soldiers, and Stone: An Introduction to Slavery in American Memory* (Washington, DC: American University), December 6, 2003, https://web.archive.org/web/20120229192309/https://www.american.edu/bgriff/dighistprojects/wym/rodney_3.htm (retrieved July 2020).

15. Jonathan W. White and Scott Sandage, "What Frederick Douglass Had to Say About Monuments," *Smithsonian*, June 30, 2020, https://www.smithsonianmag.com/history/what-frederick-douglass-had-say-about-monuments-180975225/.

16. Aishvarya Kavi, "Activists Push for Removal of Statue of Freed Slave Kneeling Before Lincoln," *New York Times*, June 27, 2020, https://www.nytimes.com/2020/06/27/us/politics/lincoln-slave-statue-emancipation.html.

17. Ibid.

18. David Lightner, "Abraham Lincoln and the Ideal of Equality," *Journal of the Illinois State Historical Society* (1908–1984) 75, no. 4 (1982): 289–308, accessed July 12, 2020, www.jstor.org/stable/40191718.

19. G. Freedman, D. N. Powell, B. Le, and K. D. Williams, "Ghosting and Destiny: Implicit Theories of Relationships Predict Beliefs about Ghosting," *Journal of Social and Personal Relationships* 36, issue 3 (2019): 905–24, https://doi.org/10.1177/0265407517748791.

20. *Harper's*, "A Letter on Justice and Open Debate," July 7, 2020, https://harpers.org/a-letter-on-justice-and-open-debate/.

21. Mary McNamara, "'Cancel Culture' Is Not the Problem: The *Harper's* Letter Is," *Los Angeles Times*, https://www.latimes.com/entertainment-arts/story/2020-07-09/cancel-culture-harpers-letter.

22. Abby Gardner, "A Complete Breakdown of the J. K. Rowling Transgender-Comments Controversy: The *Harry Potter* Author Is Being Criticized for

Comments She Made about the Trans Community," *Glamour*, July 6, 3030, https://www.glamour.com/story/a-complete-breakdown-of-the-jk-rowling-transgender-comments-controversy; for salutary tools, see Carol Tavris, "The Gadfly: Define Your Terms (Or, Here We Go Again)," *Skeptic* (Altadena, CA) 24, no. 1 (2019): 6+ (Gale Academic OneFile, accessed July 15, 2020).

23. Encyclopedia.com, "Fort-Da," Cengage, https://www.encyclopedia.com/psychology/dictionaries-thesauruses-pictures-and-press-releases/fort-da.

9. CONSPIRACY

1. Brandy Zadrozny, "Coronavirus Conspiracy Video Spreads on Instagram among Black Celebrities," NBC News, April 13, 2020, https://www.nbcnews.com/tech/social-media/coronavirus-conspiracy-video-spreads-instagram-among-black-celebrities-n1158571.

2. Ryan Bort, "Confused Republican Louie Gohmert Wonders If Wearing a Mask Led to Positive COVID Test," *Rolling Stone*, https://www.rollingstone.com/politics/politics-news/louie-gohmert-tests-positive-covid-1035799/.

3. John Locke, *An Essay Concerning Human Understanding*, Book II, chapter xxvii, "Of Identity and Diversity," sec. 8, https://enlightenment.supersaturated.com/johnlocke/BOOKIIChapterXXVII.html.

4. Martin Parker, "Conspiracies Do Exist, and This Elite Conference Is One of Them," *Quartz*, June 11, 2016, https://qz.com/704177/conspiracies-do-exist-and-this-elite-conference-is-one-of-them/.

5. Van Jones, "Opinion," CNN, April 6, 2020, https://www.cnn.com/2020/04/06/opinions/african-americans-covid-19-risk-jones/index.html.

6. FDA, "Fraudulent Coronavirus Disease 2019 (COVID-19) Products," https://www.fda.gov/consumers/health-fraud-scams/fraudulent-coronavirus-disease-2019-covid-19-products.

7. Wikipedia, "List of Unproven Methods against COVID-19," August 8, 2020, https://en.wikipedia.org/wiki/List_of_unproven_methods_against_COVID-19.

8. Jennifer A. Dlouhy, "EPA Tells Amazon, eBay to Stop Shipping Unproven COVID Goods," *Bloomberg News*, June 11, 2020, https://www.bloomberg.com/news/articles/2020-06-11/epa-orders-amazon-ebay-to-stop-shipping-unproven-covid-products.

9. Jennifer L. W. Fink, "How Hospitals Treat COVID-19 Patients," *Healthgrades*, June 16, 2020, https://www.healthgrades.com/right-care/coronavirus/how-hospitals-treat-covid-19-patients.

10. See Felix Bast, "A Nobel Laureate Said the New Coronavirus Was Made in a Lab: He's Wrong," Science, *The Wire*, April 22, 2020; Flora Teoh,

"Nobel Laureate Luc Montagnier Inaccurately Claims That the Novel Corona-virus Is Man-Made and Contains Genetic Material from HIV," Science Feed-back, Gilmore Health News, April 20, 2020, https://sciencefeedback.co/claimreview/claim-by-nobel-laureate-luc-montagnier-that-the-novel-coronavirus-is-man-made-and-contains-genetic-material-from-hiv-is-inaccurate/.

11. Mark Walker, "Scenes from a Bike Rally, Undaunted by the Virus," *New York Times*, August 9, 2020, https://www.nytimes.com/2020/08/09/us/sturgis-motorcycle.html.

12. Konstantinos Farsalinos et al., "Editorial: Nicotine and SARS-CoV-2: COVID-19 May Be a Disease of the Nicotinic Cholinergic System," Toxicology Reports, Elsevier, April 30, 2020, https://www.sciencedirect.com/science/article/pii/S2214750020302924?via%3Dihub.

13. Jeffrey Drope, "What We Know about Tobacco Use and COVID-19," American Cancer Society, April 16, 2020, https://www.cancer.org/health-care-professionals/center-for-tobacco-control/what-we-know-about-tobacco-use-and-covid-19.html.

14. Simone J. Smith, "The Corona Conspiracy; Interview with David Icke on London Real," *Toronto Caribbean*, April 14, 2020, https://torontocaribbean.com/the-corona-conspiracy-interview-with-david-icke-on-london-real/.

15. Cliff Roth, "Is 60 GHz Home Video Networking Safe?" *Electronic Engineering Times*, August 30, 2007, https://www.eetimes.com/is-60-ghz-home-video-networking-safe/.

16. Myrtill Simkó and Mats-Olof Mattsson, "5G Wireless Communication and Health Effects: A Pragmatic Review Based on Available Studies Regarding 6 to 100 GHz," *International Journal of Environmental Research and Public Health* 16, issue 18 (2019): 3406, https://www.mdpi.com/1660-4601/16/18/3406.

17. Jack Goodman and Flora Carmichael, "Coronavirus: 5G and Microchip Conspiracies around the World," *BBC Reality Check*, BBC News, June 27, 2020, https://www.bbc.com/news/53191523.

18. John Oliver, "Conspiracy Theories," *Last Week Tonight*, July 19, 2020, https://www.youtube.com/watch?v=0b_eHBZLM6U.

19. Shona Ghosh, "Conspiracy Theorists on Facebook Linking 5G to CO-VID-19 Have Now Started Pushing Hydroxychloroquine as a Virus Cure," *Business Insider*, April 10, 2020, https://www.businessinsider.com/facebook-conspiracy-group-linking-5g-to-coronavirus-also-pushes-hydroxychloroquine-2020-4.

20. Elizabeth Cohen and Wesley Bruer, "US Stockpile Stuck with 63 Million Doses of Hydroxychloroquine," CNN, June 17, 2020, https://www.cnn.com/2020/06/17/health/hydroxychloroquine-national-stockpile/index.html.

21. US Food and Drug Administration (FDA), "Coronavirus (COVID-19) Update: FDA Revokes Emergency Use Authorization for Chloroquine and Hydroxychloroquine," June 15, 2020, https://www.fda.gov/news-events/press-announcements/coronavirus-covid-19-update-fda-revokes-emergency-use-authorization-chloroquine-and.

22. Veronica Stracqualursi, "Trump Promotes a Doctor Who Has Claimed Alien DNA Was Used in Medical Treatments," CNN, July 29, 2020, https://www.cnn.com/2020/07/29/politics/stella-immanuel-trump-doctor/index.html.

23. Darlene Superville and Amanda Seitz, "Trump Defends Decision to Retweet Viral Video That Promotes Disproved Use of Malaria Drug as Treatment for COVID-19," *Chicago Tribune* /Associated Press, July 28, 2020, https:/ /www.chicagotribune.com/coronavirus/ct-nw-trump-hydroxychloroquine-video-retweet-20200728-lmhsggqh3jcjppd5ej5f2tnpvy-story.html.

24. Christi Carras, "Instagram Deletes Madonna's Post That Spread CO-VID-19 Conspiracy Theories," *Los Angeles Times*, July 29, 2020, https://www.latimes.com/entertainment-arts/music/story/2020-07-29/covid-19-madonna-instagram-video-misinformation.

25. Mark Jarrett, MD, "Will the Anti-Vaccine Community Endanger Public Health Again?" *Northwell Health*, June 29, 2020, https://www.northwell.edu/coronavirus-covid-19/news/insights/will-the-anti-vaccine-community-endanger-public-health-again-.

26. *Plandemic* (video, accessed May 9, 2020, but repeatedly taken down and difficult to find), https://www.youtube.com/watch?v=TWpjc1QZg84.

27. Kent Heckenlively and Judy Mikovits, *Plague: One Scientist's Intrepid Search for the Truth about Human Retroviruses and Chronic Fatigue Syndrome (ME/CFS), Autism, and Other Diseases* (Kindle Edition, 2014/2017; Simon & Schuster Digital Sales Inc., 2020).

28. See Davey Alba, "Virus Conspiracists Elevate a New Champion: A Video Showcasing Baseless Arguments by Dr. Judy Mikovits, Including Attacks on Dr. Anthony Fauci, Has Been Viewed More Than Eight Million Times in the Past Week," *New York Times*, May 9, 2020, https://www.nytimes.com/2020/05/09/technology/plandemic-judy-mikovitz-coronavirus-disinformation.html.

29. For Dr. Mike's comments, see "Doctor Fact-Checks Plandemic Conspiracy," YouTube, May 10, 2020, https://www.youtube.com/watch?v=TWpjc1QZg84. Dr. Mike wrote and said, "Hundreds of you have requested that I watch and respond to the *Plandemic* movie ft. Dr. Judy Mikovits, recently published on social media. I decided to check it out and respond point by point to the biggest claims the conspiracy theory movie makes. Please be respectful in the comments as the goal is to have a fruitful discussion."

30. See *Advisory Board*, "Why America Is Probably Undercounting Coronavirus Deaths," April 20, 2020, https://www.advisory.com/daily-briefing/2020/04/20/covid-count; Philip Bump, "Fauci Puts It Bluntly: Coronavirus Deaths Are Undercounted," *Washington Post*, May 20, 2020, https://www.washingtonpost.com/politics/2020/05/12/fauci-puts-it-bluntly-coronavirus-deaths-are-undercounted/.

31. Asia Ewart, "Why Doctors Are Using an Antacid to Treat Hundreds of Coronavirus Patients," *Refinery 29*, April 27, 2020, https://www.refinery29.com/en-us/2020/04/9745043/pepcid-coronavirus-heartburn-drug-treatment.

32. Davey Alba, "Virus Conspiracists Elevate a New Champion," *New York Times*, May 9, 2020, https://www.nytimes.com/2020/05/09/technology/plandemic-judy-mikovitz-coronavirus-disinformation.html.

33. Lillian Rizzo, "Sinclair Pulls Controversial Show about Coronavirus Facebook," *Wall Street Journal*, July 27, 2020, https://www.wsj.com/articles/sinclair-pulls-controversial-show-about-coronavirus-11595895808.

34. Jason Kindrachuk, "A Virologist Explains Why It Is Unlikely COVID-19 Escaped from a Lab," *Forbes*, April 17, 2020, https://www.forbes.com/sites/coronavirusfrontlines/2020/04/17/a-virologist-explains-why-it-is-unlikely-covid-19-escaped-from-a-lab/#12655bf33042.

35. Julie Bosman, "Amid Virus Surge, Republicans Abruptly Urge Masks Despite Trump's Resistance," *New York Times*, July 1, 2020, https://www.nytimes.com/2020/07/01/us/coronavirus-masks.html.

36. Colleen Curry and Alison Durkee, "Most Americans Think U.S. Is Handling Coronavirus Worse Than Other Countries—Despite Trump's Claims," *Forbes*, August 4, 2020, https://www.forbes.com/sites/colleencurry/2020/08/04/most-americans-think-us-is-handling-coronavirus-worse-than-other-countries-despite-trumps-claims/#55d76980595a.

37. Logically Fallacious, "Appeal to Authority," https://www.logicallyfallacious.com/logicalfallacies/Appeal-to-Authority.

38. See Naomi Zack, *Progressive Anonymity: From Identity Politics to Evidence-Based Government* (Lanham, MD: Rowman & Littlefield, 2020), chapters 5 and 6.

39. Tom Porter, "QAnon, the Far-Right, and Some Left-Wingers Are All Spreading Conspiracies about Trump's COVID-19 Diagnosis," *Business Insider*, October 2, 2020, https://www.businessinsider.com/qanon-plus-some-progressives-spread-trump-virus-conspiracy-theories-2020-10.

40. Gary Hart, "How Powerful Is the President? It Is Time for Congress to Investigate the Emergency Authorities Given to the Chief Executive," Opinion, *New York Times*, July 23, 2020, https://www.nytimes.com/2020/07/23/opinion/trump-presidential-powers.html.

41. Emily Badger, "How Trump's Use of Federal Forces in Cities Differs from Past Presidents," *New York Times*, July 23, 2020, https://www.nytimes.com/2020/07/23/upshot/trump-portland.html.

42. Elizabeth Thomas, "Citing Crime, Trump Expands Sending Federal Agents to Cities over Mayors' Opposition," ABC News, July 22, 2020, https://abcnews.go.com/Politics/citing-crime-trump-expand-sending-federal-agents-cities/story?id=71920102.

43. Sarah Evanega, Mark Lynas, Jordan Adams, and Karinne Smolenyak, "Coronavirus Misinformation: Quantifying Sources and Themes in the COVID-19 'Infodemic,'" Cornell Alliance for Science, Department of Global Development, Cornell University, Ithaca, New York, July 23, 2020, https://int.nyt.com/data/documenttools/evanega-et-al-coronavirus-misinformation-submitted-07-23-20-1/080839ac0c22bca8/full.pdf.

44. Annalisa Merelli, "Tracking the $5.1 Billion the US Has Spent on CO-VID-19 Medical Research," *Quartz*, July 9, 2020, https://qz.com/1877928/the-us-has-invested-over-5-billion-in-covid-19-medical-rd/.

45. See Naomi Zack, *Reviving the Social Compact: Inclusive Citizenship in an Age of Extreme Politics* (Lanham, MD: Rowman & Littlefield), chapter 6, "Natural Disaster in Society," 97–114, and chapter 7, "Environmental Disaster," 115–30.

10. ETHICS OF COVID-19 AND CLIMATE CHANGE

1. *Twisted Sifter*, "California, 1918, During 2nd Wave of Spanish Flu: 'Wear a Mask or Go to Jail,'" July 14, 2020, https://twistedsifter.com/2020/07/wear-a-mask-or-go-to-jail-spanish-flu-1918-california/.

2. James Taylor, "Wheat Production Sets New Records Thanks to Global Warming," *Forbes*, December 26, 2014, https://www.forbes.com/sites/jamestaylor/2015/02/09/top-10-global-warming-lies-that-may-shock-you/#7464d91253a5.

3. Paul Davies, "30 of the Most Impactful Climate Change Quotes," Celebrity Climate Change Quotes, *Curious Earth*, October 31, 2019, https://www.curious.earth/blog/climate-change-quotes.

4. Kathy Kinlaw and Robert Levine, "Ethical Guidelines in Pandemic Influenza," CDC, February 15, 2007, https://stacks.cdc.gov/view/cdc/11431.

5. See Naomi Zack, *Ethics for Disaster* (Lanham, MD: Rowman & Littlefield, 2009, 2010/2011); idem, "Ethics of Disaster Planning," *Philosophy of Management*, Special Issue, *Ethics of Crisis*, Per Sandin, ed., vol. 8, no. 2 (2009): 53–64.

6. Devan Cole, "Fauci Admits Earlier COVID-19 Mitigation Efforts Would Have Saved More American Lives," CNN News, April 12, 2020, https://www.cnn.com/2020/04/12/politics/anthony-fauci-pushback-coronavirus-measures-cnntv/index.html.

7. Zack, *Ethics for Disaster*, 53–64.

8. Maureen Dowd, "Double, Double, Trump's Toil, Our Trouble: Demon Sperm Meets Alien D.N.A., as President Trump Teeters," *New York Times*, August 1, 2020, https://www.nytimes.com/2020/08/01/opinion/sunday/trump-coronavirus-herman-cain.html.

9. CDC, "COVID-19 Planning Scenarios," July 10, 2020, https://www.cdc.gov/coronavirus/2019-ncov/hcp/planning-scenarios.html.

10. Becky Little, "'Mask Slackers' and 'Deadly' Spit: The 1918 Flu Campaigns to Shame People into Following New Rules," *History*, July 17, 2020, https://www.history.com/news/1918-pandemic-public-health-campaigns.

11. CDC, "CDC Takes Action to Prepare Against 'G4' Swine Flu Viruses in China with Pandemic Potential," July 2, 2020, https://www.cdc.gov/flu/spotlights/2019-2020/cdc-prepare-swine-flu.html.

12. "Small Droplet Aerosols in Poorly Ventilated Spaces and SARS-CoV-2 Transmission," Commentary, *The Lancet* 8 (July 2020), www.thelancet.com/respiratory, https://www.thelancet.com/pdfs/journals/lanres/PIIS2213-2600(20)30245-9.pdf.

13. David M. Morens and Joel G. Breman, "Coming to Terms with the Real Bioterrorist behind COVID-19: Nature," First Opinion, *STAT*, September 9, 2020, https://www.statnews.com/2020/09/09/emerging-viruses-real-bioterrorists-behind-covid-19/?utm_source=STAT+Newsletters&utm_campaign=9a08c58a5d-First_Opinion&utm_medium=email&utm_term=0_8cab1d7961-9a08c58a5d-152255802.

14. "Pandemic-Proofing the Planet: New Diseases Are Inevitable; Ensuing Global Calamities Are Not," Science & Technology, Global Health, *The Economist*, June 25, 2020, https://www.economist.com/science-and-technology/2020/06/25/pandemic-proofing-the-planet.

15. Victoria Knight, "Obama Team Left Pandemic Playbook for Trump Administration, Officials Confirm," Kaiser Health News, PBS, May 15, 2020, https://www.pbs.org/newshour/nation/obama-team-left-pandemic-playbook-for-trump-administration-officials-confirm.

16. Lev Facher, "The Coronavirus Outbreak Has Left Medical Supplies in Short Supply," *STAT*, March 10, 2020, https://www.statnews.com/2020/03/10/coronavirus-strategic-national-stockpile/.

17. Kennedy Space Center, "*Crew Dragon* Splashdown: Astronauts Bob and Doug Homecoming," August 2, 2020, https://www.kennedyspacecenter.

com/launches-and-events/events-calendar/2020/august/crew-dragon-splashdown.

18. See James Hansen, "Climate Change in a Nutshell: The Gathering Storm," Columbia.com, December 18, 2018, http://www.columbia.edu/~jehl/mailings/2018/20181206_Nutshell.pdf; US Environmental Protection Agency (EPA), "Overview of Greenhouse Gases," Greenhouse Gas Emissions, https://www.epa.gov/ghgemissions/overview-greenhouse-gases.

19. Climate Nexus, "Animal Agriculture's Impact on Climate Change," https://climatenexus.org/climate-issues/food/animal-agricultures-impact-on-climate-change/.

20. E. U. Weber, "Experience--Based and Description-Based Perceptions of Long--Term Risk: Why Global Warming Does Not Scare Us (Yet)," *Climatic Change* 77 (2006): 103–20, https://www.researchgate.net/publication/226378293_Experience-Based_and_Description-Based_Perceptions_of_Long-Term_Risk_Why_Global_Warming_Does_Not_Scare_Us_Yet.

21. John Foster, *After Sustainability: Denial, Hope, Retrieval* (New York: Routledge, 2015), 24.

22. F. C. S. Schiller, "Aristotle and the Practical Syllogism," *Journal of Philosophy, Psychology and Scientific Methods* 14, no. 24 (November 22, 1917): 645–53, http://www.jstor.com/stable/2940162.

23. Anthony Leiserowitz, Edward Maibach, Seth Rosenthal, and John Kotcher, *Climate Change in the American Mind*, 19ff, Yale Climate Change Communication and George Mason University, Center for Climate Change Communication, April 2020, https://climatecommunication.yale.edu/wp-content/uploads/2020/05/climate-change-american-mind-april-2020b.pdf.

24. George Singleton, "Akrasia: Why Do We Act Against Our Better Judgement?" Free Will, *Philosophy Now,* 2016, https://philosophynow.org/issues/112/Akrasia_Why_Do_We_Act_Against_Our_Better_Judgement.

25. See Ross Douthat, "The Age of Decadence," Opinion, *New York Times*, February 7, 2020, https://www.nytimes.com/2020/02/07/opinion/sunday/western-society-decadence.html; idem, *The Decadent Society: How We Became Victims of Our Own Success* (New York: Simon & Schuster, 2020).

26. Andrew Freedman, Jason Samenow, Kim Bellware, and Emily Wax-Thibodeaux, "Western Wildfires: Evacuations in California and Oregon as Destructive Fire Outbreak Engulfs Region," *Washington Post*, September 9, 2020, https://www.washingtonpost.com/weather/2020/09/09/western-fires-live-updates/.

27. Tania Schoennagel, Jennifer K. Balch, Hannah Brenkert-Smith, Philip E. Dennison, Brian J. Harvey, Meg A. Krawchuk, Nathan Mietkiewicz, Penelope Morgan, Max A. Moritz, Ray Rasker, Monica G. Turner, and Cathy Whitlock, "Adapt to Wildfire as Climate Changes," *Proceedings of the National*

Academy of Sciences 114, no. 18 (May 2017): 4582–90, DOI: 10.1073/
pnas.1617464114; Volker C. Radeloff, David P. Helmers, H. Anu Kramer,
Miranda H. Mockrin, Patricia M. Alexandre, Avi Bar-Massada, Van Butsic,
Todd J. Hawbaker, Sebastián Martinuzzi, Alexandra D. Syphard, Susan I.
Stewart, "Rapid Growth of the US Wildland-Urban Interface Raises Wildfire
Risk," *Proceedings of the National Academy of Sciences* 115, no. 13 (March
2018): 3314–19, DOI: 10.1073/pnas.1718850115.

28. Caroline Kelly, "LA Mayor on Trump's Response to Wildfires: 'This Is
Climate Change,' Not Just about Forest Management," CNN, September 13,
2020, https://www.cnn.com/2020/09/13/politics/west-coast-fires-eric-garcetti-
climate-change-cnntv/index.html.

29. Harvard T. H. Chan School of Public Health, "Coronavirus, Climate
Change, and the Environment: A Conversation on COVID-19 with Dr. Aaron
Bernstein, Director of Harvard Chan C-CHANGE," consulted for update on
August 6, 2020, https://www.hsph.harvard.edu/c-change/subtopics/
coronavirus-and-climate-change/.

30. Susan Arbetter, "Cuomo: $3 Billion New York Environmental Bond Act
Postponed," New York State, Spectrum News NY1, New York City, July 30,
2020, https://www.ny1.com/nyc/all-boroughs/ny-state-of-politics/2020/07/30/
cuomo---3-billion-new-york-environmental-bond-act-postponed.

31. Zack Colman, "CFTC Report: Climate Change Poses Serious Risk to
Financial System," *Politico*, September 8, 2020, https://www.politico.com/
news/2020/09/08/cftc-report-climate-change-poses-serious-risk-to-financial-
system-410573; Coral Davenport and Jeanna Smialek, "Federal Report Warns
of Financial Havoc from Climate Change," *New York Times*, September 9,
2020, https://www.nytimes.com/2020/09/08/climate/climate-change-financial-
markets.html.

CONCLUSION

1. See Naomi Zack, *Progressive Anonymity: From Identity Politics to Evidence-Based Government* (Lanham, MD: Rowman & Littlefield, 2020).

2. Irwin Redlener, MD; Jeffrey D. Sachs, PhD; Sean Hansen, MPA; Nathaniel Hupert, MD, "130,000–210,000 Avoidable COVID-19 Deaths—and
Counting—in the U.S.," National Center for Disaster Preparedness, Columbia
University, October 21, 2020, https://ncdp.columbia.edu/custom-content/
uploads/2020/10/Avoidable-COVID-19-Deaths-US-NCDP.pdf.

3. Prabhash K. Dutta, "New Virus Found in China, Another Pandemic
Feared: Is Yet Another Pandemic Coming?" *India Today*, June 30, 2020,

https://www.indiatoday.in/science/story/new-virus-in-china-another-pandemic-feared-1695395-2020-06-30.

4. CDC, "CDC Takes Action to Prepare Against 'G4' Swine Flu Viruses in China with Pandemic Potential," July 2, 2020, https://www.cdc.gov/flu/spotlights/2019-2020/cdc-prepare-swine-flu.html.

5. Slavoj Žižek, *Pandemic! COVID-19 Shakes the World* (New York: OR Books, LLC/Polity Press, 2020), 44, 129–31.

6. John Locke, *An Essay Concerning Human Understanding*, edited by Peter H. Nidditch (Oxford: Oxford University Press, 1690/1975), book II, chapter xxi, section 10, 238.

7. Benjamin Hart, "Trump Supporters Left Stranded in Cold after Omaha Rally," *Intelligencer*, *New York Magazine*, October 28, 2020, https://nymag.com/intelligencer/2020/10/trump-supporters-left-stranded-in-cold-after-omaha-rally.html.

SELECT BIBLIOGRAPHY

POPULAR AND GENERAL SOURCES

ABC News. https://abcnews.go.com/.
American Cancer Society. https://www.cancer.org/.
American Psychological Association. https://www.apa.org/.
Arizona Republic. https://www.azcentral.com/.
Associated Press. https://apnews.com/f4988865f4fad739e099b17707f8727f.
The Atlantic. https://www.theatlantic.com/.
Barron's. https://www.barrons.com/.
BBC News. https://www.bbc.com/news/.
Bloomberg News. https://www.bloomberg.com/news/.
Brookings. https://www.brookings.edu/blog/.
BuzzFeed News. https://www.buzzfeednews.com/.
CBS News. http://www.cbsnews.com/news/.
Center for Disability Studies. https://www.cds.udel.edu/.
Chicago Tribune. https://www.chicagotribune.com/.
CNBC. https://www.cnbc.com/.
CNN News. https://www.cnn.com/.
College Tuition Compare. http://blog.collegetuitioncompare.com.
Computer Hope. https://www.computerhope.com/.
Com/Talk, College of Communication, Boston University. https://www.bu.edu/com/comtalk.
The Conversation. https://theconversation.com/.
Courthouse News Service. https://www.courthousenews.com/.
Daily Mail. https://www.dailymail.co.uk/news.
The Economist. https://www.economist.com.
Education Week. "The Coronavirus Spring: The Historic Closing of U.S. Schools, July 1, 2020." https://www.edweek.org/ew/section/multimedia/the-coronavirus-spring-the-historic-closing-of.html.
Electronic Engineering Times. https://www.eetimes.com/.
Elemental. Medium. https://elemental.medium.com/.
Elon University News. https://www.elon.edu/u/news/.
Federal Safety Net. http://federalsafetynet.com/us-poverty-statistics.html.
Forbes. https://www.forbes.com/.
FOX Business. https://www.foxbusiness.com/.
Glamour. https://www.glamour.com/.
Global Citizen. https://www.globalcitizen.org/.

The Guardian. https://www.theguardian.com.
Harper's magazine. https://harpers.org.
Harvard Business Review, August 19, 2016. https://hbr.org/.
Harvard Gazette. https://news.harvard.edu/gazette/.
Healthgrades. https://www.healthgrades.com/.
The Hill. June 12, 2020. https://thehill.com/.
History. https://www.history.com/.
India Today. https://www.indiatoday.
Intelligencer. *New York Magazine*. https://nymag.com/intelligencer/.
Investing Answers. https://investinganswers.com/dictionary/.
Investopedia. https://www.investopedia.com/.
Kaiser Family Foundation (KFF). https://www.kff.org/.
Knowledia. https://news.knowledia.com/.
Lakota Times. https://www.lakotatimes.com/.
Logically Fallacious. https://www.logicallyfallacious.com/.
lohud.com. New York State Team. https://www.lohud.com/story/news/.
Los Angeles Times. https://www.latimes.com/.
Marketplace. https://www.marketplace.org/.
MarketWatch. https://www.marketwatch.com/.
Médecins Sans Frontières. https://www.doctorswithoutborders.org/covid19; idem, USA. https://www.doctorswithoutborders.org/what-we-do/news-stories/news/msf-helps-respond-needs-vulnerable-communities-us-during-covid-19.
Medicine Net. https://www.medicinenet.com/.
National Council on Aging (NCOA). "COVID-19 Resources for Older Adults & Caregivers." https://www.ncoa.org/ncoa_acf/covid-19-resources-for-older-adults/.
National Public Radio (NPR). https://www.npr.org/.
NBC News. https://www.nbcnews.com/.
New Europe. https://www.neweurope.eu/.
New Yorker. https://www.newyorker.com/.
New York Post. https://nypost.com/.
New York Region, *New York Times*. https://www.nytimes.com/.
New York Times. https://www.nytimes.com/.
New York Times Magazine. https://www.nytimes.com/2020/06/25/magazine/.
Norton Internet Security. https://us.norton.com/internetsecurity.
Pew Research Center. https://www.pewresearch.org/fact-tank/.
Phys.org. https://phys.org/news/.
Politico. https://www.politico.com/news/.
PolitiFact. The Poynter Institute. https://www.politifact.com/.
Psychology Today. https://www.psychologytoday.com/.
Quartz. https://qz.com/.
Radio.com. https://www.radio.com/news/.
Real Clear Politics. https://www.realclearpolitics.com/.
Reason. https://reason.com/.
Refinery 29. https://www.refinery29.com/en-us/.
Reform Austin. https://www.reformaustin.org/.
Reuters, May 2020. https://www.reuters.com/.
Rolling Stone. https://www.rollingstone.com/.
Safety Detectives. https://www.safetydetectives.com/blog/antivirus-statistics/.
Sapiens. https://www.sapiens.org/.
ScienceDaily. www.sciencedaily.com/.
ScienceDirect. https://www.sciencedirect.com.
Smithsonian magazine. https://www.smithsonianmag.com/.
South China Morning Post (SCMP.org). https://www.scmp.com/news/china/article/.
Spectrum News NY1, New York City. https://www.ny1.com/nyc/.
STAT. https://www.statnews.com/.
tctMD, June 10, 2020. https://www.tctmd.com/.

The Telegraph. https://www.telegraph.co.uk/.
Texas Tribune. https://www.texastribune.org/.
Time. https://time.com/.
Toofab. https://toofab.com/.
Toronto Caribbean. https://torontocaribbean.com/.
Twisted Sifter. https://twistedsifter.com/.
Twitter. https://twitter.com/.
UCSF News. https://www.ucsf.edu/.
Vanity Fair. https://www.vanityfair.com/.
Wall Street Journal. https://www.wsj.com/.
Washington Post. https://www.washingtonpost.com/.
Washington Times. https://www.washingtontimes.com/.
Westwood One Podcasts. http://www.westwoodonepodcasts.com/pods/the-prof-g-show-with-scott-galloway/.
WIRED. https://www.wired.com/.
YouTube. https://www.youtube.com/.

FILM AND VIDEO

Dr. Mike's comments on *Plandemic*: "Doctor Fact-Checks Plandemic Conspiracy." YouTube, May 10, 2020. https://www.youtube.com/watch?v=TWpjc1QZg84.
The Godfather: Part II. https://www.youtube.com/watch?v=DfHJDLoGInM.
"Inside Italy's War on COVID" (Documentary). *Frontline*, season 20, episode 19, PBS, March 19, 2020. https://www.pbs.org/wgbh/frontline/film/inside-italys-covid-war/.
Network. Metro-Goldwyn-Mayer, 1976. https://www.imdb.com/title/tt0074958/.
Oliver, John. "Conspiracy Theories." *LastWeekTonight*, July 19, 2020. https://www.youtube.com/watch?v=0b_eHBZLM6U.
Plandemic (video). Accessed May 9, 2020, but repeatedly taken down and difficult to find. https://www.youtube.com/watch?v=TWpjc1QZg84.

OFFICIAL SOURCES AND REFERENCES

American Academy of Pediatrics. https://www.aappublications.org/.
American College Health Association (ACHA). https://www.acha.org/.
Brennan Center for Justice. https://www.brennancenter.org/.
Bureau of Economic Analysis (BEA). https://www.bea.gov/.
Center for Infectious Disease Research and Policies (CIDRAP). https://www.cidrap.umn.edu/covid-19/supply-chain-issues.
Center for the Study of Federalism. https://encyclopedia.federalism.org/.
Centers for Disease Control and Prevention (CDC). https://www.cdc.gov/.
———. "COVID-19." https://www.cdc.gov/coronavirus/.
Climate Nexus. "Animal Agriculture's Impact on Climate Change." https://climatenexus.org/climate-issues/food/animal-agricultures-impact-on-climate-change/.
Department of Homeland Security. https://www.dhs.gov/.
Econofact. https://econofact.org/.
Emergency Management Assistance Compact (EMAC). The All Hazards National Mutual Aid System. https://www.emacweb.org/.
Encyclopedia Britannica. https://www.britannica.com/.
Federal Emergency Management Administration (FEMA). https://www.fema.gov/.
Federal News Network. https://federalnewsnetwork.com/government-news/.
Food and Drug Administration (FDA). https://www.fda.gov/.

Kennedy Space Center. https://www.kennedyspacecenter.com/.

Lawfare, March 14, 2020. https://www.lawfareblog.com/.

Legal Information Institute, Cornell Law School. https://www.law.cornell.edu/constitution/amendmentxxv.

National Center for Education Statistics. "Back to School Statistics," "Educational," Fast Facts. https://nces.ed.gov/fastfacts/.

National Conference of State Legislatures. https://www.ncsl.org/.

National Governors' Association (NGA). https://www.nga.org/policy-communications/letters-nga/.

National Humanities Center. http://nationalhumanitiescenter.org/.

National Law Enforcement Officers Memorial Fund. https://nleomf.org/facts-figures/law-enforcement-facts.

National Library of Medicine, National Institutes of Health. "Disaster Health Information Sources: The Basics." Disaster Information, Management Resource Center. https://www.nlm.nih.gov/dis_courses/basics/01-000.html.

New York State Government. COVID-19 Updates. https://coronavirus.health.ny.gov/.

———. Childcare Services, Office of Family Services. https://ocfs.ny.gov/programs/childcare/.

Organization for Economic Co-operation and Development (OECD). https://www.oecd.org/unitedstates/.

Pew Research Center. https://www.pewresearch.org/fact-tank/.

Siblis Research. "Total Market Value of U.S. Stock Market." June 30, 2020. https://siblisresearch.com/data/.

Trading Economics. https://tradingeconomics.com/.

US Department of Labor, Bureau of Labor Statistics. https://www.bls.gov/.

White House. Coronavirus Task Force. https://www.whitehouse.gov/briefings-statements/.

———. Health Care. https://www.whitehouse.gov/briefings-statements/.

World, Real Matters/WNG.org. https://world.wng.org/.

LEGAL CASES

Graham v. Connor, 490 U.S. 389 (1989). https://en.wikipedia.org/wiki/Graham_v._Connor.

Plumhoff et al. v. Rickard, US Supreme Court, October Term, 2013. http://www.supremecourt.gov/opinions/13pdf/12-1117_1bn5.pdf.

Tennessee v. Garner, 471 U.S. 1 (1985). *FindLaw*, 7–12. http://caselaw.lp.findlaw.com/scripts/getcase.pl?court=US&vol=471&invol=1.

Terry v. Ohio. 392 I/S/ 1(1968), no. 67. http://scholar.google.com/scholar_case?case=17773604035873288886&q=terry+v.+ohio,+us+supreme+court&hl=en&as_sdt=3,38.

SCHOLARLY, ACADEMIC, AND PROFESSIONAL SOURCES

Abbasi, Jennifer. "Taking a Closer Look at COVID-19, Health Inequities, and Racism." *JAMA Network* 324, no. 5 (2020): 427–29. DOI:10.1001/jama.2020.11672, https://jamanetwork.com/journals/jama/fullarticle/2767948.

Abramovitz, Mimi. "Economic Crises, Neoliberalism, and the US Welfare State: Trends, Outcomes and Political Struggle." In *Global Social Work: Crossing Borders, Blurring Boundaries*, 225–40. In Carolyn Noble, Helle Strauss, and Brian Littlechild, eds. Australia: Sydney University Press, 2014. Accessed August 26, 2020. http://www.jstor.org/stable/j.ctv1fxm2q.20.

Abramson, Jerry. "10 Cities Making Real Progress since the Launch of the 21st Century Policing Task Force." White House/President Barack Obama, May 18, 2015. https://

obamawhitehouse.archives.gov/blog/2015/05/18/10-cities-making-real-progress-launch-21st-century-policing-task-force.

Adams, Richard E., William M. Rohe, and Thomas A. Arcury. "Implementing Community-Oriented Policing: Organizational Change and Street Officer Attitudes." *Crime and Delinquency*, July 1, 2002. https://doi.org/10.1177/0011128702048003003, https://journals.sagepub.com/doi/abs/10.1177/0011128702048003003.

Ahmed, N., S. Thompson, and M. Glaser. "Global Aquaculture Productivity, Environmental Sustainability, and Climate Change Adaptability." *Environmental Management* 63 (2019): 159–72. https://doi.org/10.1007/s00267-018-1117-3.

Alexander, Michelle. *The New Jim Crow: Mass Incarceration in the Age of Colorblindness.* New York: New Press, Kindle Edition, 2012.

Anderson, Tricia, Frederic Levy, Michael Wagner, and Ryan Burnette. "State of Emergency: COVID-19, the Stafford Act, and What It All Means for Contractors." Posted in Coronavirus, COVID-19, Government Contracts Regulatory Compliance, State and Local Procurements, March 18, 2020. https://www.insidegovernmentcontracts.com/2020/03/state-of-emergency-COVID-19-the-stafford-act-and-what-it-all-means-for-contractors/.

Ariès, Philippe. *Centuries of Childhood.* Trans. Robert Baldick. New York: Alfred A. Knopf, 1962.

Bahle, Thomas. "Public Child Care in Europe: Historical Trajectories and New Directions." In K. Scheiwe and H. Willekens, eds., *Childcare and Preschool Development in Europe*, 23–42. London: Palgrave Macmillan, 2009.

Berman, Emily. "The Roles of the State and Federal Government in a Pandemic." *Journal of National Security Law & Policy* (2020). Available at SSRN: https://ssrn.com/abstract=3617058 or http://dx.doi.org/10.2139/ssrn.3617058 (accessed June 27, 2020).

Bittner, E. "Quasi-Military Organization of Police." In Victor E. Kappeler, ed., *Police and Society: Touchstone Readings*, 173–84. National Criminal Justice Reference Service (NCJRS), NCJ-151401, 1995. https://www.ncjrs.gov/App/Publications/abstract.aspx?ID=151410.

Breen, Richard. "Education and Intergenerational Social Mobility in the US and Four European Countries." *Oxford Review of Economic Policy* 35, issue 3 (Autumn 2019): 445–66. https://doi.org/10.1093/oxrep/grz013.

Caldara, R., and L. Vizioli. "The Speed of Race" [Abstract]. *Journal of Vision* 10, issue 7 (2010): 699, 699a. http://www.journalofvision.org/content/10/7/699. DOI:10.1167/10.7.699.

Centers for Disease Control and Prevention. "CDC Takes Action to Prepare Against 'G4' Swine Flu Viruses in China with Pandemic Potential." July 2, 2020. https://www.cdc.gov/flu/spotlights/2019-2020/cdc-prepare-swine-flu.html.

Coates, Ta-Nehisi. *Between the World and Me.* New York: Random House, 2015.

Colman, Zack. "CFTC Report: Climate Change Poses Serious Risk to Financial System." *Politico*, September 8, 2020. https://www.politico.com/news/2020/09/08/cftc-report-climate-change-poses-serious-risk-to-financial-system-410573.

Cunningham, Jamein, and Rob Gillezeau. "Don't Shoot! The Impact of Historical African American Protest on Police Killings of Civilians." *Journal of Quantitative Criminology* (2019): 1–34. 10.1007/s10940-019-09443-8.

Davies, Margaret. "Home and State: Reflections on Metaphor and Practice." *Griffith Law Review* 23, issue 2 (2014): 153–75. DOI: 10.1080/10383441.2014.962447.

Dew, Charles B. *Apostles of Disunion: Southern Secession Commissioners and the Causes of the Civil War.* Charlottesville: University of Virginia Press, 2001/2017.

Dewey, John. *Moral Principles in Education, II: The Moral Training Given by the School Community.* Chicago, IL: Houghton Mifflin, 1909. http://catalog.lambertvillelibrary.org/texts/American/dewey/moral/moral.htm. DOI: 10.1126/science.abb2762.

Douthat, Ross. *The Decadent Society: How We Became Victims of Our Own Success.* New York: Simon & Schuster, 2020.

Dunn, Gibson. "The Constitutional Consequences of Governmental Responses to COVID-19: The Right to Travel and the Dormant Commerce Clause." May 1, 2020. https://www.

gibsondunn.com/the-constitutional-consequences-of-governmental-responses-to-COVID-19-the-right-to-travel-and-the-dormant-commerce-clause/.

Dynes, Russell R. "The Dialogue between Voltaire and Rousseau on the Lisbon Earthquake: The Emergence of a Social Science View." Disaster Research Center, 1999. http://udspace.udel.edu/handle/19716/435.

El-Masri, Souheil, and Graham Tipple. "Natural Disaster, Mitigation and Sustainability: The Case of Developing Countries." *International Planning Studies* 7, issue 2 (2002): 157–75. DOI: 10.1080/13563470220132236.

Evanega, Sarah, Mark Lynas, Jordan Adams, and Karinne Smolenyak. "Coronavirus Misinformation: Quantifying Sources and Themes in the COVID-19 'Infodemic.'" Cornell Alliance for Science, Department of Global Development. Cornell University, Ithaca, New York, July 23, 2020. https://int.nyt.com/data/documenttools/evanega-et-al-coronavirus-misinformation-submitted-07-23-20-1/080839ac0c22bca8/full.pdf.

Farsalinos, Konstantinos, et al. "Editorial: Nicotine and SARS-CoV-2: COVID-19 May Be a Disease of the Nicotinic Cholinergic System." Toxicology Reports, *Elsevier*, April 30, 2020. https://www.sciencedirect.com/science/article/pii/S2214750020302924?via%3Dihub.

Foster, John. *After Sustainability: Denial, Hope, Retrieval.* New York: Routledge, 2015.

Freedman, G., D. N. Powell, B. Le, and K. D. Williams. "Ghosting and Destiny: Implicit Theories of Relationships Predict Beliefs about Ghosting." *Journal of Social and Personal Relationships* 36, issue 3 (2019): 905–24. https://doi.org/10.1177/0265407517748791.

Fritz, Charles E. "Disasters." In Robert K. Merton and Robert A. Nisbet, eds., *Contemporary Social Problems*, 651–94. New York: Harcourt, 1961.

Hansen, James. "Climate Change in a Nutshell: The Gathering Storm." Columbia.com, December 18, 2018. http://www.columbia.edu/~jeh1/mailings/2018/20181206_Nutshell.pdf.

Harvard T. H. Chan School of Public Health. "Coronavirus, Climate Change, and the Environment: A Conversation on COVID-19 with Dr. Aaron Bernstein, Director of Harvard Chan C-CHANGE." Consulted for update on August 6, 2020. https://www.hsph.harvard.edu/c-change/subtopics/coronavirus-and-climate-change/.

Heckenlively, Kent, and Judy Mikovits. *Plague: One Scientist's Intrepid Search for the Truth about Human Retroviruses and Chronic Fatigue Syndrome (ME/CFS), Autism, and Other Diseases.* Kindle Edition (2014/2017), Simon & Schuster Digital Sales Inc., 2020.

Hildebrand, David L. *Dewey: A Beginner's Guide.* Oxford: One World Books, 2008 (from John Dewey, "Between Two Worlds," 1944, LW17: 463). https://epdf.pub/queue/dewey-a-beginners-guide-beginners-guide-oneworld.html.

Hockett, Robert, and Aaron James. *Money from Nothing: Or, Why We Should Stop Worrying about Debt and Learn to Love the Federal Reserve.* New York: Melville House, 2020.

Holt, Douglas B. "Does Cultural Capital Structure American Consumption?" *Journal of Consumer Research* 25, issue 1 (June 1998): 1–25. https://doi.org/10.1086/209523.

Hume, David. "Of Justice." In *An Inquiry Concerning the Principles of Morals*, 22–23. Indianapolis, IN: Hackett, 1983. Also at *An Inquiry Concerning the Principles of Morals.* Project Gutenberg, Section III, "Of Justice," Part III, "Justice." https://www.gutenberg.org/files/4320/4320-h/4320-h.htm.

Ioanide, Paula. *The Emotional Politics of Racism: How Feelings Trump Facts in an Era of Colorblindness.* Stanford, CA: Stanford University Press, 2015.

Jarrett, Mark. "Will the Anti-Vaccine Community Endanger Public Health Again?" Northwell Health, June 29, 2020. https://www.northwell.edu/coronavirus-covid-19/news/insights/will-the-anti-vaccine-community-endanger-public-health-again-.

Kinlaw, Kathy, and Robert Levine. "Ethical Guidelines in Pandemic Influenza." CDC, February 15, 2007. https://stacks.cdc.gov/view/cdc/11431.

Klein, Naomi. *The Shock Doctrine: The Rise of Disaster Capitalism.* New York: Henry Holt, 2008.

Knight, Victoria. "Obama Team Left Pandemic Playbook for Trump Administration, Officials Confirm." Kaiser Health News, PBS, May 15, 2020. https://www.pbs.org/newshour/nation/obama-team-left-pandemic-playbook-for-trump-administration-officials-confirm.

Kraemer, M. U. G., A. Sadilek, Q. Zhang, et al. "Mapping Global Variation in Human Mobility." *Nature Human Behaviour* (2020). https://doi.org/10.1038/s41562-020-0875-0.

Kupferschmidt, Kai. "'A Completely New Culture of Doing Research': Coronavirus Outbreak Changes How Scientists Communicate." *Science*, February 26, 2020. https://www.sciencemag.org/news/2020/02/completely-new-culture-doing-research-coronavirus-outbreak-changes-how-scientists.

Lawrence, Sarah, and Bobby McCarthy. "What Works in Community Policing." Chief Justice Earl Warren Institute on Law and Social Policy, University of California, Berkeley School of Law, November 2013. https://www.law.berkeley.edu/files/What_Works_in_Community_Policing.pdf.

Leeb, R. T., S. Price, S. Sliwa, et al. "COVID-19 Trends among School-Aged Children: United States, March 1–September 19, 2020." *Morbidity and Mortality Weekly Report* (CDC) 69 (2020): 1410–15. DOI: http://dx.doi.org/10.15585/mmwr.mm6939e2, https://www.cdc.gov/mmwr/volumes/69/wr/mm6939e2.htm#suggestedcitation.

Leigh, Robert D., ed. *A Free and Responsible Press: A General Report on Mass Communication: Newspapers, Motion Pictures, Radio, Magazines, and Books, by the Commission on Freedom of the Press.* Chicago and London: University of Chicago Press, 1947/Midway Press, 1974.

Leiserowitz, Anthony, Edward Maibach, Seth Rosenthal, and John Kotcher. *Climate Change in the American Mind.* Yale Climate Change Communication and George Mason University, Center for Climate Change Communication, April 2020. https://climatecommunication.yale.edu/wp-content/uploads/2020/05/climate-change-american-mind-april-2020b.pdf.

Levin, Janet. "Functionalism." In Edward N. Zalta, ed., *Stanford Encyclopedia of Philosophy* (Fall 2018). https://plato.stanford.edu/archives/fall2018/entries/functionalism/.

Lightner, David. "Abraham Lincoln and the Ideal of Equality." *Journal of the Illinois State Historical Society* (1908–1984) 75, no. 4 (1982): 289–308. Accessed July 12, 2020. www.jstor.org/stable/40191718.

Locke, John. *An Essay Concerning Human Understanding*, book II, chapter xxvii, "Of Identity and Diversity," sec. 8. https://enlightenment.supersaturated.com/johnlocke/BOOKIIChapterXXVII.html/.

———. *An Essay Concerning Human Understanding.* Edited by Peter H. Nidditch. Oxford: Oxford University Press, 1690/1975.

———. "Some Considerations of the Consequences of the Lowering of Interest and Rising the Value of Money." In Patrick Hyde Kelly, ed., *Locke on Money*, vol. 1. Oxford: Oxford Clarendon Press, 1991.

Lu, R., X. Zhao, J. Li, P. Niu, B. Yang, H. Wu, et al. "Genomic Characterisation and Epidemiology of 2019 Novel Coronavirus: Implications for Virus Origins and Receptor Binding." *The Lancet* 395, issue 10224 (February 2020): 565–74.

Martini, M., V. Gazzaniga, N. L. Bragazzi, and I. Barberis. "The Spanish Influenza Pandemic: A Lesson from History 100 Years after 1918." *Journal of Preventive Medicine and Hygiene* 60, no. 1 (March 29, 2019): E64–E67. DOI:10.15167/2421-4248/jpmh2019.60.1.1205, https://www.ncbi.nlm.nih.gov/pmc/articles/PMC6477554/.

Mill, John Stuart. *On Liberty.* Excerpts, *OpenMind Platform*, 22. http://openmindplatform.org/wp-content/uploads/2018/02/John-Stuart-Mill_On-Liberty_Excerpts.pdf.

Mirowsky, John, and Catherine E. Ross. *Education, Social Status, and Health.* New York: Routledge, 2003.

Monahan, Torin. "Securing the Homeland: Torture, Preparedness, and the Right to Let Die." *Social Justice* 33, no. 1 (2006): 95–105. https://publicsurveillance.com/papers/Securing_the_Homeland.pdf.

Mullin, John R. "The Reconstruction of Lisbon Following the Earthquake of 1755: A Study in Despotic Planning." *Journal of the International History of City Planning Association* (1992): 45. https://scholarworks.umass.edu/larp_faculty_pubs/45.

Myers, K. R, W. Y. Tham, Y. Yin, et al. "Unequal Effects of the COVID-19 Pandemic on Scientists." *Nature Human Behaviour*, July 15, 2020. https://doi.org/10.1038/s41562-020-0921-y, https://www.nature.com/articles/s41562-020-0921-y.

Nagel, Thomas. "Moral Luck." In *Mortal Questions*, 24–38. Cambridge, MA: Cambridge University Press, 1979.

Newmyer, Kent. "*John Marshall McCulloch v. Maryland* and the Southern States' Rights Tradition." *John Marshall Law Review* 33, issue 4 (2000): 875–934.

Nielsen, Kai. "Against Moral Conservativism." *Ethics* 82, no. 3 (1972): 219–31.

Nietzsche, Friedrich. "Reason in Philosophy," Sec. 1, *Twilight of the Idols: Or How to Philosophize with the Hammer*, trans. Richard Polt. Indianapolis, IN: Hackett, 1997/2009.

Núñez, Amber Colón. "The Coronavirus Crisis Is Capitalism in Action: Here's How the Left Can Respond." *In These Times*, March 27, 2020. https://inthesetimes.com/article/coronavirus-crisis-capitalism-naomi-klein-covid-19.

Nyamutata, Conrad. "Do Civil Liberties Really Matter During Pandemics? Approaches to Coronavirus Disease (COVID-19)." *International Human Rights Law Review* 9, issue 1 (May 24, 2020): 62–98. https://brill.com/view/journals/hrlr/9/1/article-p62_62.xml.

Padala, P. R., A. M. Jendro, and K. P. Padala. "Conducting Clinical Research during the COVID-19 Pandemic: Investigator and Participant Perspectives." *JMIR Public Health Surveillance* 6, no. 2 (April 6, 2020): e18887. DOI:10.2196/18887, https://www.ncbi.nlm.nih.gov/pmc/articles/PMC7141248/.

Piketty, Thomas. *Capital in the Twenty-First Century*. Trans. Arthur Goldhammer. Cambridge, MA: Harvard University Press, 2014.

Privitera, Greta. "Italian Doctors on Coronavirus Frontline Face Tough Calls on Whom to Save." Politico.eu, March 9, 2020. https://www.politico.eu/article/coronavirus-italy-doctors-tough-calls-survival/.

Quarantelli, E. L. "What Is Disaster? The Need for Clarification in Definition and Conceptualization in Research." Disaster Research Center, University of Delaware, Research, Series Report, Article 177 (1985): 41–73. http://udspace.udel.edu/handle/19716/1119.

Quarantelli, E. L., P. Lagadec, and A. Boin. "A Heuristic Approach to Future Disasters and Crises: New, Old, and In-Between Types." In E. L. Quarantelli, ed., *Handbook of Disaster Research*. Handbooks of Sociology and Social Research. New York: Springer, 2007.

Radeloff, Volker C., David P. Helmers, H. Anu Kramer, Miranda H. Mockrin, Patricia M. Alexandre, Avi Bar-Massada, Van Butsic, Todd J. Hawbaker, Sebastián Martinuzzi, Alexandra D. Syphard, and Susan I. Stewart. "Rapid Growth of the US Wildland-Urban Interface Raises Wildfire Risk." *Proceedings of the National Academy of Sciences* 115, no. 13 (March 27, 2018): 3314–19. DOI: 10.1073/pnas.1718850115.

Robson, Ruthann. "Positive Constitutionalism in a Pandemic: Demanding Responsibility from the Trump Administration." *ConLawNOW* 12, issue 1 (2020): 15. https://ideaexchange.uakron.edu/conlawnow/vol12/iss1/2/.

Rozell, Mark J., and Clyde Wilcox. *Federalism: A Very Short Introduction*. New York: Oxford University Press, 2019.

Saloner, Brendan, Kalind Parish, Julie A. Ward, et al. "COVID-19 Cases and Deaths in Federal and State Prisons." *JAMA Network*, July 8, 2020. https://jamanetwork.com/journals/jama/fullarticle/2768249.

Schiller, F. C. S. "Aristotle and the Practical Syllogism." *Journal of Philosophy, Psychology and Scientific Methods* 14, no. 24 (November 22, 1917): 645–53.

Schoennagel, Tania, Jennifer K. Balch, Hannah Brenkert-Smith, Philip E. Dennison, Brian J. Harvey, Meg A. Krawchuk, Nathan Mietkiewicz, Penelope Morgan, Max A. Moritz, Ray Rasker, Monica G. Turner, and Cathy Whitlock. "Adapt to Wildfire as Climate Changes." *Proceedings of the National Academy of Sciences* 114, no. 18 (May 2017): 4582–90. DOI: 10.1073/pnas.1617464114.

Simkó, Myrtill, and Mats-Olof Mattsson. "5G Wireless Communication and Health Effects: A Pragmatic Review Based on Available Studies Regarding 6 to 100 GHz." *International Journal of Environmental Research and Public Health* 16, issue 18 (2019): 3406. https://www.mdpi.com/1660-4601/16/18/3406.

Singleton, George. "Akrasia: Why Do We Act Against Our Better Judgement?" Free Will, *Philosophy Now* (2016). https://philosophynow.org/issues/112/Akrasia_Why_Do_We_Act_Against_Our_Better_Judgement.

"Small Droplet Aerosols in Poorly Ventilated Spaces and SARS-CoV-2 Transmission." Commentary, *The Lancet* 8 (July 2020). www.thelancet.com/respiratory, https://www.thelancet.com/pdfs/journals/lanres/PIIS2213-2600(20)30245-9.pdf.

Tabarrok, Alex. "A Pandemic Trust Fund." COVID Recovery Symposium, April 2020. https://www.thecgo.org/wp-content/uploads/2020/04/Pandemic-Trust-Fund.pdf.

Tavris, Carol. "The Gadfly: Define Your Terms (Or, Here We Go Again)." *Skeptic* (Altadena, CA) 24, no. 1 (2019): 6+. Gale Academic OneFile, accessed July 15, 2020.

Taylor, Keeanga-Yamahtta. "How Do We Change America: The Quest to Transform This Country Cannot Be Limited to Challenging Its Brutal Police." *Blackpast*, "(1951) We Charge Genocide," July 15, 2011. https://www.blackpast.org/global-african-history/primary-documents-global-african-history/we-charge-genocide-historic-petition-united-nations-relief-crime-united-states-government-against/.

Timmerman, Travis. "A Case for Removing Confederate Monuments." In Bob Fischer, ed., *Ethics, Left and Right: The Moral Issues That Divide Us*, 513–22. New York: Oxford University Press, 2020. https://philpapers.org/archive/TIMACF.pdf.

Trump, Mary L., PhD. *Too Much and Never Enough: How My Family Created the World's Most Dangerous Man*. New York, London: Simon & Schuster, 2020.

US Department of Agriculture, Food and Nutrition Service. "Find Meals for Kids When Schools Are Closed." https://www.fns.usda.gov/meals4kids.

US Environmental Protection Agency (EPA). "Overview of Greenhouse Gases." Greenhouse Gas Emissions. https://www.epa.gov/ghgemissions/overview-greenhouse-gases.

Wallace, Bob. "Medical Innovations: From the 1918 Pandemic to a Flu Vaccine." National World War II Museum, April 13, 2020. https://www.nationalww2museum.org/war/articles/medical-innovations-1918-flu.

Wan, William, Carolyn Y. Johnson, and Joel Achenbach. "States Rushing to Reopen Are Likely Making a Deadly Error, Coronavirus Models and Experts Warn." *Washington Post*, April 22, 2020. https://www.washingtonpost.com/health/2020/04/22/reopening-america-states-coronavirus/.

Weber, E. U. "Experience-Based and Description-Based Perceptions of Long-Term Risk: Why Global Warming Does Not Scare Us (Yet)." *Climatic Change* 77 (2006): 103–20. 10.1007/s10584-006-9060-3.

White, Jonathan W., and Scott Sandage. "What Frederick Douglass Had to Say about Monuments." *Smithsonian* magazine, June 30, 2020. https://www.smithsonianmag.com/history/what-frederick-douglass-had-say-about-monuments-180975225/.

Wigginton, N. S., R. M. Cunningham, R. H. Katz, M. E. Lidstrom, K. A. Moler, D. Wirtz, M. T. Zuber. "Moving Academic Research Forward during COVID-19." *Science* 368, issue 6496 (June 12, 2020): 1190–92. DOI: 10.1126/science.abc5599.

Woodward, Bob. *Rage*. New York: Simon & Schuster, 2020.

Yan, Renhong, Yuanyuan Zhang, Yaning Li, Lu Xia, Yingying Gou, and Qiang Zhou. "Structural Basis for the Recognition of SARS-CoV-2 by Full-Length Human ACE2." *Science* 367, issue 6485 (March 27, 2020): 1444–48. https://science.sciencemag.org/content/367/6485/1444.

Yancy, Clyde W. "COVID-19 and African Americans." *JAMA Network*, April 15, 2020. https://jamanetwork.com/journals/jama/fullarticle/2764789.

Young, Rodney A. "Great Emancipator, Supplicant Slave: The Freedman's Memorial to Abraham Lincoln." *Slaves, Soldiers, and Stone: An Introduction to Slavery in American Memory*. Washington, DC: American University, December 6, 2003. https://web.archive.org/web/20120229192309/https://www.american.edu/bgriff/dighistprojects/wym/rodney_3.htm (retrieved July 2020).

Zack, Naomi. "The Big Question with Naomi Zack." *Scientific Inquirer*, May 27, 2020. https://scientificinquirer.com/2020/05/27/the-big-question-with-naomi-zack-ethics-and-the-covid-19-pandemic/.

———. *Ethics for Disaster*. Lanham, MD: Rowman & Littlefield, 2009, 2010/2011.

———. "Ethics of Disaster Planning." *Philosophy of Management*. Special Issue, "Ethics of Crisis," Per Sandin, ed., vol. 8, no. 2 (2009): 53–64.

———. "Lockean Money, Globalism and Indigenism." In Catherine Wilson, ed., "Civilization and Oppression." *Canadian Journal of Philosophy* 25 (1999): 31–53.

———, ed. *Oxford Handbook of Philosophy and Race.* New York: Oxford University Press, 2017.

———. "Philosophy and Disaster." *Homeland Security Affairs Journal* 2, issue 1, article 5 (April 2006). https://www.hsaj.org/articles/176.

———. *Philosophy of Race: An Introduction.* New York: Palgrave Macmillan, Springer, 2018.

———. *Progressive Anonymity: From Identity Politics to Evidence-Based Government.* Lanham, MD: Rowman & Littlefield, 2020.

———. *Reviving the Social Compact: Inclusive Citizenship in an Age of Extreme Politics.* Lanham, MD: Rowman & Littlefield, 2018.

———. "Suffrage Comes with Obligations. Voting Is Only the First." *Forward*, August 18, 2020. https://forward.com/culture/452827/suffrage-obligations-voting-only-the-first-19th-amendment-centennial/.

———. *White Privilege and Black Rights: The Injustice of U.S. Police Racial Profiling and Homicide.* Lanham, MD: Rowman & Littlefield, 2015.

Žižek, Slavoj. *Pandemic! COVID-19 Shakes the World.* New York: OR Books, LLC/Polity Press, 2020.

Zwick, Rebecca. "Assessment in American Higher Education: The Role of Admissions Tests." *The Annals of the American Academy of Political and Social Sciences*, May 16, 2019. https://journals.sagepub.com/doi/abs/10.1177/0002716219843469.

INDEX

ABOUT THE AUTHOR

Naomi Zack, PhD, Columbia University, has been professor of philosophy at Lehman College, CUNY, since 2019. She earlier taught at SUNY, Albany, and at the University of Oregon. Her most recent book is *Progressive Anonymity: From Identity Politics to Evidence-Based Government*. Additional books include *Reviving the Social Compact: Inclusive Citizenship in an Age of Extreme Politics* (2018), her edited fifty-one-essay *Oxford Handbook of Philosophy and Race* (2017), *Philosophy of Race: An Introduction* (2018), *The Theory of Applicative Justice: An Empirical Pragmatic Approach to Correcting Racial Injustice* (2016), *White Privilege and Black Rights: The Injustice of U.S. Police Racial Profiling and Homicide* (2015), *The Ethics and Mores of Race: Equality after the History of Philosophy* (2011/2015), *Ethics for Disaster* (2009, 2010–2011), *Inclusive Feminism: A Third Wave Theory of Women's Commonality* (2005), *Philosophy of Science and Race* (2002), and *Race and Mixed Race* (1992). In progress is *Democracy*, a VSI (Very Short Introduction) in the Oxford University Press series. Naomi Zack was awarded the Romanell–Phi Beta Kappa Professorship for 2019–2020, with lectures to be given on the Lehman campus, which were delayed due to COVID-19 lockdowns in New York City. She will be giving the John Dewey Lecture at the Pacific Division Meeting of the American Philosophical Society in April 2021. She has been teaching an online course, "Disaster and Corona," at Lehman College.